UNDERSTANDING DEMENTIA CAREGIVER CHALLENGES:

---

10 STEPS TO NAVIGATE SYMPTOMS, OVERCOME DAILY CHALLENGES, AND CREATE A CALM ENVIRONMENT, EVEN IF YOU FEEL LOST.

DEAN RAMSEY

CONTENTS

❦ Created with Vellum

DEDICATION

Dedication

This book is lovingly dedicated to Agnes and Paul, my parents, who suffered from this. To my wife, Devie, a special thanks for her endless patience, understanding, and love. Her steadfast presence and wise counsel have made this journey possible and easier. Thank you for being by my side through every word and every challenge. Your belief in me transforms the impossible into reality. And a special thank you to all the caregivers over the years who helped make their lives a little better and brighter and their days a little easier when I couldn't be there.

INTRODUCTION

In the quiet moments of the night, when the world seems to hold its breath, the reality of being a caregiver to someone with dementia can feel overwhelmingly complex. Every day is a challenging journey, requiring the caregiver's skills, attention, trust, and connection with the patient to provide the best care possible. This book, "Understanding Dementia Caregiver Challenges," was born from a deep desire to cast a light on this path—offering hope, understanding, and practical guidance to those who walk it daily. I aim to create a sanctuary within these pages where caregivers feel recognized, understood, and far from alone. Here, in the shared stories and strategies, we find common ground and collective strength.

My connection to dementia caregiving is not as an outsider looking in but as someone who has lived through the highs and lows that define this journey. This personal experience has fueled my passion and grounded my approach in reality, empathy, and a profound respect for those who face these challenges daily. This perspective sets this book apart, making it more than just a guide; it will be your companion.

This book is structured around ten critical steps designed to guide you through the essential aspects of dementia caregiving. From understanding symptoms to overcoming daily hurdles and fostering a peaceful environment, each chapter builds on the last, offering practical advice, real-life insights, and emotional support. Within these pages, innovative caregiving strategies are combined with stories from caregivers like you, all underscored by a focus on resilience, self-care, and the indomitable spirit of those who give so much of themselves.

To the incredible adults aged 25-45 who balance the demands of caregiving with countless other life responsibilities, this book is for you. You are neither alone in feeling the weight of this role nor in your moments of doubt and exhaustion. Here, you will find strategies, insights, validation, and encouragement that acknowledge your unique challenges and contributions.

I invite you, then, to not just read this book but to engage with it. Reflect on your own experiences, draw from the insights shared, and apply them in ways that resonate with your journey. This is an opportunity to join a community of caregivers, to share in the wisdom gathered here, and to find your own path through the complexities of dementia caregiving.

Let us conclude this introduction with a note of hope and empowerment. Despite the undeniable challenges ahead, it is entirely possible to navigate dementia caregiving with resilience, finding moments of joy and meaning along the way. Together, let us step forward into this journey equipped with the knowledge, strategies, and compassion this book offers. Herein lies the promise of surviving and thriving in the role of a dementia caregiver.

CHAPTER 1

THE ROAD TO DEMENTIA CARE

"The greatest gift you can give to someone is your time, your attention, your love, your concern." - Joel Osteen.

I n the heart of a bustling city, under the soft glow of the streetlamps, a man in his late sixties walks home, his steps uncertain, his mind clouded. He might appear merely lost or deep in thought to the casual observer. However, his reality is one that millions across the globe share—a life altered by dementia. The illness is generally characterized by forgetfulness, loss of memory, and a general cognitive decline.

This condition, often misunderstood and shrouded in myths, significantly impacts not just those diagnosed but also their families and caregivers. It's not merely a story of forgotten names and lost keys but a profound shift in the cognitive fabric that defines our humanity. Therefore, it is imperative to understand its nuanced nature and how one may navigate dementia's complexities.

Understanding Dementia's True Nature

Dementia is not a single illness but a term that encompasses a spectrum of neurological conditions affecting cognitive functions such as memory, thinking, orientation, comprehension, calculation, learning capacity, language, and judgment. The World Health Organization (WHO) describes it as a syndrome—usually of a chronic or progressive nature—in which there is deterioration in cognitive function beyond what might be expected from the usual consequences of biological aging. It is crucial to distinguish dementia from the minor memory lapses that can occur with normal aging, as dementia significantly impairs social and occupational functioning.

Types of Dementia

The various forms of dementia, including Alzheimer's disease, vascular dementia, Lewy body dementia, and frontotemporal dementia, each affect the brain in different ways. Alzheimer's disease, the most common type of dementia, involves the parts of the brain that control thought, memory, and language. Vascular dementia, often resulting from stroke or other conditions affecting blood flow to the brain, impacts problem-solving and focus. Lewy body dementia is characterized by abnormal protein deposits in the brain, leading to thinking, movement, behavior, and mood issues. Frontotemporal dementia affects the frontal and temporal lobes of the brain, influencing personality, behavior, and language. Each type presents its own set of challenges, symptoms, and progression patterns, underscoring the complexity of dementia as a whole.

At the core of dementia's impact is the disruption of brain function. Neurodegenerative diseases like Alzheimer's involve the buildup of proteins such as beta-amyloid plaques and tau tangles, leading to the death of nerve cells and the loss of brain tissue. In vascular dementia, brain damage is often due to conditions that block or reduce blood flow to the brain, depriving brain cells of the oxygen and nutrients they need to function effectively. The changes in brain chemistry and structure directly correlate with the symptoms observed in dementia, from memory lapses and confusion to difficulty with speech and changes in personality.

Misconceptions about Dementia

Despite its prevalence, numerous myths surround dementia. One common misconception is that it is an inevitable part of aging. While age is the most potent known risk factor for dementia, it is not a normal part of aging. Many people live into their 90s and beyond without any signs of dementia. Another widespread myth is that dementia solely affects memory. While memory loss is a common symptom, especially in the early stages of Alzheimer's, dementia can also impair reasoning, judgment, language, and other cognitive abilities. It's this multifaceted impact that makes dementia particularly challenging for individuals and their families.

For caregivers and loved ones, gaining a deeper insight into the nature of dementia, its varied forms, and the brain chemistry involved is the first step toward providing compassionate and practical support. By dispelling myths and embracing the multifaceted reality of dementia, we can begin to comprehend the illness with the sensitivity and awareness that is needed to ensure that those affected by dementia continue to live with dignity and a sense of connection to the world around them.

Emotional Landscape: Empathy First

The realm of emotions surrounding dementia is vast and varied, affecting both the individual with the condition and their caregivers. Recognizing and responding to these emotions with empathy is crucial in fostering meaningful connections and effective communication.

Emotional Toll on the Individual

For someone living with dementia, the world can become a confusing, sometimes frightening place. Imagine waking up one day to find familiar faces and places suddenly strange and unrecognizable. This confusion often leads to frustration, as simple tasks that once came naturally now present insurmountable challenges. Fear is another common emotion stemming from losing control over one's environment and faculties. Individuals might also experience sadness as they sense their memories and abilities slipping away, mourning the loss of their former selves. Recognizing these emotions is the first step towards empathetic care, allowing caregivers to see beyond the symptoms of dementia and connect with the person experiencing them.

Caregiver Emotions

Caregivers traverse their emotional landscape. Guilt is a frequent companion, arising from impatience, frustration, or simply believing they could always do more. There is also the profound sadness of watching a loved one fade away, coupled with a sense of loss for the shared memories that no longer resonate with the person they're caring for. Amid these challenging emotions, caregivers might find moments of joy and connection, which become precious oases in the desert of caregiving. These emotional highs and lows underscore the need for emotional intelligence in caregiving—recognizing, understanding, and managing one's emotions and the emotions of the person with dementia.

Building Empathy

Cultivating empathy begins with stepping into the shoes of the person with dementia, striving to understand their world and how they perceive it. Although it is impossible in such situations to create a level of relatability, some strategies can help one enhance empathy:

- Active Listening: Pay close attention to what is being said and left unsaid. Observe body language and facial expressions to understand their feelings and needs better.
- Patience: Allow them the time to express themselves, understanding that their thought processes may be slower.

- Validation: Acknowledge their feelings and experiences as authentic and valid. Even if their perceptions may not align with reality, it is their reality, and it's essential to validate that.
- Learning: Invest time in learning about dementia and its impact on both cognitive and emotional levels. This knowledge can foster a deeper understanding of the challenges faced by the individual.

Empathetic Conversations

Empathy shapes not only our thoughts but also how we communicate. Communicating with empathy ensures clarity in your conversations, which helps to build trust and feelings of security between the caregiver and the patient. Here are some tips for empathetic communication:

- Simplify Your Speech: Use simple, clear sentences and avoid open-ended questions that could confuse or overwhelm the listener. Instead of asking, "What would you like for lunch?" you might say, "Would you like soup for lunch?"
- Non-verbal Cues: Much of our communication is non-verbal. Maintain eye contact, use gentle touches, and ensure your body language is open and approachable to convey your message effectively.
- Reassurance: Individuals with dementia might feel insecure or anxious. Offer reassurance through your words and actions, reinforcing that they are in a safe space.
- Distraction and Redirection: If they become upset or agitated, gently redirect their attention to a different topic or activity they enjoy. This can help alleviate stress and bring comfort.

Empathy serves as a bridge, connecting the world of dementia with the reality of caregiving. It's about seeing the person, not the disease; understanding their emotions, fears, and frustrations; and communicating in a way that respects and honors their individuality.

Through empathy, caregivers can forge deeper connections, making each interaction more meaningful and supportive.

Beyond Memory Loss: Dementia's Diverse Symptoms

When most people think of dementia, memory loss is often the first symptom that comes to mind. However, the condition's reach extends beyond forgetting names or misplacing items. It encompasses a range of cognitive, psychological, and physical symptoms that can affect nearly every aspect of daily life. Understanding the full spectrum of symptoms not only aids in early detection but also informs better management strategies for those living with the condition.

Cognitive Symptoms

Dementia's impact on cognition goes well beyond memory lapses. We must understand that dementia is a loss of cognitive and executive functions that humans take for granted. Brains damaged in dementia cannot perform everyday thinking, decision-making, critical thinking, and other brain functions. Individuals may encounter significant challenges with:

- Problem-Solving: Tasks that require planning, sequencing, dealing with numbers, and abstract thinking can become notably tricky. This might manifest in managing finances, following a recipe, or planning an outing.
- Complex Tasks: Multistep activities such as driving, cooking, or managing medications may become overwhelming due to the inability to focus on multiple elements simultaneously.
- Language: Finding the right words becomes a struggle, affecting speech and comprehension. Conversations can be frustrating when words are on the tip of the tongue but refuse to come forth.
- Orientation: Time and place can become confusing concepts. An individual might lose track of dates, seasons, or even the

passage of time during the day, leading to disorientation even in familiar environments.

These cognitive challenges often lead to a noticeable decline in the ability to perform daily activities independently, signaling a need for increased care and support.

Psychological Changes

The psychological impact of dementia can be as varied and complex as its cognitive symptoms. However, this brings to light the need for a holistic approach to dementia care, addressing mental and emotional health alongside physical and cognitive needs. There can be various changes in the behavior of a patient with dementia, including the following:

- Mood Swings: Rapid, unexplained changes in mood, from calm to tears or anger, can occur without apparent reason. These swings can be distressing for the individual and their caregivers, adding an unpredictable element to daily care.
- Personality Changes: Significant alterations in personality might manifest, with individuals becoming more withdrawn, suspicious, irritable, or aggressive. These changes are particularly challenging as they may contrast sharply with the person's pre-dementia demeanor.
- Depressive Episodes: Depression is not uncommon, characterized by sustained periods of sadness, withdrawal from social activities, loss of interest in previously enjoyed hobbies, and changes in appetite or sleep patterns.

Physical Effects

While the cognitive and psychological symptoms of dementia are more widely recognized, the condition can also have a profound impact on the bodies of those suffering from it. Let's have a look at a few more apparent physical effects of dementia:

- Coordination Problems: Challenges with coordination and motor functions can emerge, affecting balance and increasing the risk of falls. Fine motor skills might also decline, such as buttoning clothes or using utensils.
- Sleep Disturbances: Individuals may experience changes in their sleep patterns, including difficulty falling asleep, staying asleep, or waking up frequently throughout the night. Day-night confusion, known as "sundowning," can exacerbate these issues, leading to increased agitation or confusion in the late afternoon and evening.
- Appetite and Weight Changes: Changes in taste, smell, and appetite can lead to unintentional weight loss or, conversely, weight gain if the individual forgets they have already eaten and consumes more food.

These physical manifestations of dementia not only affect the individual's quality of life but also pose significant challenges for caregivers in managing daily care routines and ensuring safety.

Early Diagnosis and Prognosis

Recognizing the diverse symptoms of dementia—beyond just memory loss—is crucial for early detection and diagnosis. Now that you are familiar with the most common overall symptoms of dementia, you are in a better position to detect it and consult a physician in time. This is significant in ensuring a better quality of life for your loved one because early detection opens the door to various benefits. These include access to treatments that may slow the progression of specific symptoms and the opportunity to plan for the future. At the same time, the individual can still participate in decision-making and implementing management strategies to improve quality of life.

Moreover, understanding the breadth of dementia's impact can help caregivers and loved ones tailor their support to address the specific challenges faced by the individual. Whether adapting communication strategies to deal with language difficulties, modifying the home environment to improve safety and reduce confusion, or seeking professional help to manage psychological symptoms, a comprehensive understanding of dementia's diverse symptoms is vital in the caregiving toolkit.

Perhaps even more important than early detection is learning about the risk factors associated with dementia. It is the same old yet effective way of thinking: prevention is better than cure. Therefore, the following section addresses how we can focus on identifying and addressing the possible causes of dementia.

Minimizing the Risks

While the exact cause of many forms of dementia remains elusive, research has identified several lifestyle factors and health conditions that can influence the risk of developing dementia. Addressing these can play a crucial role in reducing one's risk. It's about making informed choices today that can benefit brain health in the long term.

Healthy Diet

A balanced diet of fruits, vegetables, lean protein, and healthy fats can support brain health. The Mediterranean diet, mainly, has been linked to a lower risk of cognitive decline. This diet emphasizes:

- Plenty of fruits and vegetables
- Whole grains
- Fish and poultry over red meat
- Olive oil as a primary fat source

Incorporating such foods into daily meals can nourish the brain and body, potentially warding off dementia.

Regular Physical Activity

Exercise is not only good for the heart but also for the brain. Regular physical activity increases blood flow to the brain, which can help maintain healthy brain function and encourage the growth of new brain cells. Aim for at least 150 minutes of moderate-intensity exercise each week, such as brisk walking, cycling, or swimming. Even incorporating more movement into daily routines, like taking the stairs instead of the elevator, can add up and contribute to brain health.

Mental Stimulation

Keeping the mind active is as crucial as physical exercise. Activities that challenge the brain – puzzles, reading, learning a new skill, or even playing musical instruments – can strengthen brain cells and their connections. Consider this as setting up a savings account for brain health; the more deposits made through mental stimulation, the richer the cognitive reserve in later years.

Social Engagement

Staying socially active can combat isolation and depression, both of which are risk factors for dementia. Regular interaction with friends, family, and community members keeps the mind engaged and can improve mood and well-being. Whether joining a club, volunteering, or simply sharing meals with others, fostering social connections is critical.

Control Heart Health

There is a strong link between cardiovascular health and brain health. Conditions that damage the heart or arteries, such as high blood pressure, high cholesterol, diabetes, and obesity, can also increase dementia risk. When necessary, managing these through diet, exercise, and medication can protect the brain and the heart.

Avoid Tobacco and Limit Alcohol

Smoking and excessive alcohol consumption are both associated with an increased risk of dementia. Quitting smoking and moderating alcohol intake can significantly reduce this risk. Support is available for those who find it challenging to quit smoking or reduce alcohol consumption, from counseling services to support groups and medical interventions.

Sleep Well

Quality sleep is vital for flushing toxins from the brain that accumulate during the day. Establishing a regular sleep schedule, creating a restful environment, and addressing sleep disorders can improve sleep quality. For those struggling with sleep, consider relaxation techniques before bed, such as reading or meditation, and limit screen time to support a healthy sleep cycle.

Manage Stress

Chronic stress can have a detrimental effect on the brain, contributing to memory problems and cognitive decline. Finding healthy ways to manage stress is essential. This might include regular exercise, meditation, deep breathing exercises, or talking things out with a trusted friend or therapist. Identifying stressors and learning coping mechanisms can protect brain health.

Regular Health Check-ups

Staying on top of general health can catch potential problems early. Regular check-ups with a healthcare provider can help manage chronic conditions like diabetes or high blood pressure before they can impact brain health. Discussing concerns about memory or cognitive function during these visits can also lead to early detection and management of potential issues.

In essence, while the risk of developing dementia cannot be eliminated, adopting a lifestyle that supports overall health can significantly reduce the risk. It's about making daily choices that benefit the body and the brain, laying a foundation for maintaining cognitive function in later life.

Neuroplasticity and Dementia Care

Neuroplasticity offers a glimmer of hope in dementia care. Neuroplasticity refers to the brain's remarkable ability to form new connections and pathways in response to learning and experience. This adaptability is not just the preserve of young, developing brains but continues throughout life. Even in the face of neurodegenerative diseases like dementia, the brain can find ways to reroute signals and create new pathways, offering opportunities for intervention and care that were once thought impossible.

Neuroplasticity shows us that the brain is not a static organ but can change and adapt. In dementia, where specific pathways become blocked or communication between neurons is lost, the brain's plastic nature means it can, to some extent, "rewire" itself to maintain functionality. This ability is at the heart of cognitive rehabilitation techniques designed to slow the progression of dementia symptoms and improve quality of life.

Cognitive Rehabilitation

Cognitive rehabilitation is a set of therapies that are aimed at restoring healthy brain function after a brain injury or in progressive neurodegenerative diseases. In dementia, it leverages neuroplasticity through targeted activities and exercises that stimulate cognitive function. These can include:

- Memory Training: Exercises designed to improve working memory and recall. This might involve mnemonics, visualization techniques, or memory aids.
- Attention and Concentration Exercises: Tasks that require focused attention, such as puzzle-solving or simple math problems, can strengthen these cognitive abilities.
- Language and Communication Activities: Engaging in conversations, storytelling, or writing exercises helps maintain language skills. For those at earlier stages of dementia, learning a new language or musical instrument can be

particularly beneficial, offering cognitive challenge and enjoyment.

- Problem-solving Tasks: Activities that require planning, reasoning, and decision-making can help keep these skills sharp. Simple daily tasks can be practical, like planning a meal or organizing a drawer.
- Incorporating these techniques into daily routines stimulates the brain and provides a sense of achievement and purpose for individuals with dementia.

Adapting to New Realities

Dementia brings with it everchanging and completely life-altering circumstances. Therefore, as dementia progresses, adapting to new realities becomes increasingly essential. Caregivers play a crucial role in this adaptation process, helping their loved ones navigate the changing landscape of their abilities while maintaining dignity and a sense of self. Strategies for adaptation include:

- Modifying the Environment: Adjusting the living space reduces confusion and enhances safety. This might involve simplifying layouts, using labels and signs, and ensuring good lighting.
- Routine and Structure: Establishing a consistent daily routine that accommodates the individual's current abilities can provide a comforting sense of predictability.
- Focus on Abilities: Emphasizing and building on what the individual can still do, rather than what they have lost, fosters a positive atmosphere and encourages engagement.
- Creative Expression: Encouraging involvement in art, music, or dance provides an outlet for emotion and self-expression that transcends verbal communication.

These adaptations not only support the person with dementia but also provide caregivers with practical strategies for managing care effectively.

Promoting Brain Health

Alongside cognitive rehabilitation, lifestyle changes and activities that promote overall brain health can play a significant role in dementia care. These include:

- Nutrition for the Brain: A diet rich in antioxidants, omega-3 fatty acids, and vitamins, similar to the Mediterranean diet, supports brain health. Incorporating foods like berries, leafy greens, nuts, and fish can help protect brain cells and promote new growth.
- Physical Exercise: Regular physical activity increases blood flow to the brain and can encourage the growth of new brain cells. Activities that combine physical and cognitive elements, such as dancing or tai chi, are especially beneficial.
- Social Connections: Maintaining social ties and engaging in meaningful social activities stimulate the brain and can improve mood and well-being.
- Mental Stimulation: Keeping the brain active through hobbies, learning new skills, or engaging in intellectually stimulating activities helps build cognitive reserve.
- Mindfulness and Relaxation: Meditation, yoga, or deep-breathing exercises reduce stress and positively affect cognitive function.

By integrating these practices into daily life, caregivers can support their loved ones in maintaining brain health and potentially slowing the progression of dementia symptoms. These strategies, grounded in the principles of neuroplasticity, offer a proactive approach to dementia care that focuses on possibility, adaptation, and resilience.

Raising Dementia Awareness

There are abundant misconceptions in dementia care, to the point that they distort the true nature of the condition. This distortion not only muddies public understanding but also affects those directly involved

—both individuals living with dementia and their caregivers. Tackling these myths head-on clears the fog of misunderstanding, paving the way for better support and care.

One pervasive myth is that dementia is a singular disease rather than a syndrome encompassing a range of conditions that impair cognitive functions. This is not as much a myth as a consequence of a lack of awareness. This simplification obscures the complexity of dementia, leading to misconceptions about its causes, symptoms, and prognosis.

Another widespread belief is that dementia symptoms are solely the result of aging and, therefore, inevitable. This not only is incorrect but also minimizes the experiences of those affected, suggesting their conditions are untreatable and hopeless. In reality, dementia results from various diseases and injuries that affect the brain, many of which can be managed with appropriate care and intervention.

The Impact of Misinformation

The myths surrounding dementia contribute significantly to the stigma and isolation experienced by individuals with the condition and their caregivers. For instance, the misconception that dementia leads to a complete loss of self can cause society to prematurely disengage from those diagnosed, treating them as if they are already gone. This stigma can discourage individuals and families from seeking diagnosis and support, fearing judgment and misunderstanding from their community. The isolation that often results from this stigma can exacerbate the challenges of dementia, leading to increased caregiver burden and diminished quality of life for those with the condition.

Misinformation about dementia has far-reaching consequences, affecting decisions about treatment, care, and even daily interactions. For example, the belief that significant memory loss is a normal part of aging may prevent early detection and treatment of dementia, denying individuals the benefit of interventions that could improve their quality of life. Similarly, the myth that people with dementia cannot benefit from social interaction or engage in meaningful activities can lead to reduced opportunities for engagement, contributing to a decline in cognitive function and emotional well-being.

Educating the Public

Combatting these myths requires a concerted effort to educate the public, fostering a more informed and compassionate community. Here are several strategies caregivers and advocates can employ:

- Information Campaigns: Utilizing social media, community newsletters, and local events to share accurate information about dementia. Infographics and bite-sized videos can be especially effective in conveying key messages.
- Personal Stories: Sharing personal stories of life with dementia can humanize the condition, breaking down stereotypes and building empathy. Whether through blog posts, community talks, or media interviews, these stories can shift perceptions and reduce stigma.
- Community Engagement: Collaborating with local schools, businesses, and organizations to host dementia awareness events. Interactive workshops that simulate the sensory and cognitive challenges faced by those with dementia can be particularly eye-opening.
- Advocacy: Engaging with policymakers and health organizations to advocate for more robust dementia education in the healthcare system and the broader community. Ensuring that professionals across sectors—from healthcare to law enforcement—are trained in dementia awareness can improve the overall response to and care for those with the condition.
- Support Networks: Creating and promoting support networks for individuals with dementia and their caregivers. These networks can provide emotional support and a platform for advocacy and public education efforts.
- Resource Sharing: Compiling and distributing lists of resources, including books, websites, and local services, that offer accurate information about dementia. Libraries,

community centers, and health clinics can be critical partners
in disseminating these resources.

In dispelling myths and spreading accurate information, we chip away
at the stigma and isolation that too often accompany a dementia
diagnosis. This not only improves the lives of those directly affected by
dementia but also creates a society that is better equipped to support
them. Through education and advocacy, we can shift the narrative
around dementia, building a foundation of understanding,
compassion, and respect.

CHAPTER 2

THE CAREGIVER'S COMPASS

"To care for those who once cared for us is one of the highest honors." - Tia Walker.

I magine the first day of a new job. There's no manual; the tasks vary by the hour, and your boss communicates in a way you're just beginning to understand. This scenario mirrors the early days of becoming a caregiver for someone with dementia. It's a role without a roadmap yet demands patience, creativity, and an enormous heart. Here, we navigate the terrain of embracing this role, from the initial challenges to finding deep, personal meaning in caregiving.

The Initial Transition

The shift from family member to caregiver often happens gradually, a subtle slide into a world of medications, appointments, and new routines. Suddenly, you're making decisions you never thought you'd have to, like managing finances or personal care for someone who once took care of you. This shift can stir emotions, from honor and love to fear and uncertainty. It can also alter family dynamics, reshuffling roles as everyone finds their footing in this new landscape. Recognizing these changes and talking openly about them can help. A family meeting, where everyone shares their thoughts and concerns, can be a good starting point. It's also a space to discuss practicalities, like who can do what and when, ensuring the care is a team effort, not a solo mission.

Identity and Self-Perception

Becoming a caregiver changes how you see yourself. Where you once identified primarily as a daughter, son, spouse, or friend, you now have this significant role that shapes your daily life. Some days, it might feel like caregiving is all you do. Yet, it's vital to remember you're more than this role. Maintaining hobbies, interests, and connections outside of caregiving helps preserve your sense of self. It might be as simple as keeping a weekly coffee date with a friend or setting aside time each day for something you love, be it reading, gardening, or just taking a quiet walk. These activities aren't selfish; they're necessary, providing a well of energy and patience to draw from in your caregiving role.

Setting Boundaries

Setting boundaries is crucial for your well-being and your ability to care effectively. It means knowing when to say no, when to ask for help, and when to take a break. Start by listing your non-negotiables, the things you need to function well, like eight hours of sleep, a daily shower, or an hour of quiet each evening. Communicate these needs to others and work together to find ways to meet them. It's also helpful to set boundaries around your time and energy. This might mean scheduling specific times for caregiving tasks, delegating where possible, and being clear about what you can and cannot do. Remember, setting boundaries isn't about pushing people away; it's about ensuring you can care for your loved one without losing yourself.

Finding Meaning

Amidst the challenges, there's a profound opportunity for meaning in the caregiving role. It's found in the small moments: a shared laugh, an old story retold, a quiet afternoon spent side by side. These moments remind us of the love and connection that underpin our caregiving efforts. They also provide a sense of purpose, a confirmation that what we're doing matters intensely. Finding meaning helps you reflect on your motivations and values. Consider keeping a journal, noting the moments of joy and fulfillment, however small. Over time, these entries paint a picture of your impact, not just in your loved one's life but also in your growth and understanding.

Finding meaning also comes from connecting with others on this path. Support groups, in-person or online, offer a space to share stories, challenges, and victories. Hearing from others in similar situations can validate your experiences and provide new perspectives on finding joy and purpose in caregiving.

Caregiving for someone with dementia is a profound act of love and courage. It reshapes lives, alters identities, and challenges us in ways we never imagined. Yet, within this role lies the potential for incredible growth, deep connection, and meaningful contributions to the lives of those we care for. As we navigate this path, remember to care for ourselves with the compassion and dedication we offer our loved ones. After all, it's in nurturing our well-being that we find the strength to meet the demands of caregiving with grace, resilience, and love.

Managing Guilt, Grief, and Anxiety

Most people who have dementia are cared for in their homes by family members or significant others. These caregivers often experience substantial psychosocial distress, including feelings of guilt, grief, and anxiety. These emotions can be overwhelming and may have a detrimental impact on the well-being of the caregiver. As the disease progresses, these feelings can become more robust, and a sense of helplessness can also set in. However, it would help if you remembered that these emotions are normal and natural responses to the challenges of caring for someone you love, who is eroding before your eyes. It is no doubt difficult. While it is crucial to acknowledge and validate these emotions, you should also seek support and resources to manage these complicated feelings.

Navigating Guilt

Guilt often shadows the steps of those caring for loved ones with dementia. It whispers doubts and fuels worries over whether enough is being done, moments of impatience signify failure, or if balancing life's other demands with caregiving duties means falling short in both arenas. To ease this burden, consider:

- Acknowledging Feelings: Admit to yourself that feeling unwell is a natural part of caregiving. It's okay to have these feelings, but it's also crucial to challenge them.
- Setting Realistic Expectations: Remind yourself that perfection is unattainable. You're doing the best you can with the resources and knowledge you have.
- Seeking Reassurance: Talk about your feelings with friends, family, or support groups. Often, they can offer the perspective and reassurance you need to see the tremendous job you're doing.
- Forgiveness: Practice forgiving yourself for any perceived shortcomings. Remind yourself of the love and effort you're putting into caregiving.

Grieving the Living

Grief doesn't wait for the end; it intertwines with dementia caregiving, mourning the loss of the person as they were. This grief is complex, ebbing and flowing as moments of clarity bring back the person you remember, only for the tide of dementia to take them away again. It can take a toll on the caregiver's personal mental health and ability to provide good care for their loved one as well. Therefore, handling this grief is necessary. It involves:

- Acknowledgment: First, you must recognize that grieving the living is valid and you feel natural emotions. It's a process that allows you to mourn the gradual changes in your loved one.
- Expressing Emotions: Allow yourself to feel and express your grief. Find a way to express sadness through tears, writing, art, or conversation.
- Cherishing Moments: Focus on making new memories with your loved one, even in the most minor ways. These moments can provide comfort and connection amidst the grief.
- Professional Support: Sometimes, grief becomes too heavy to carry alone. Therapists or counselors specialized in grief can offer strategies and support to navigate these feelings.

Anxiety and Uncertainty

Anxiety often accompanies caregiving, fueled by concerns for what the future holds and the health of your loved one. The uncertainty of progression, the worry about providing adequate care, and the fear of what's to come can be overwhelming. Anxiety can be disorienting and even scary; it can bring you down into a state of strange paranoia, anticipating the worst. However, seeing it as it is again essential: a natural response to a gradual loss. You can deal with anxiety better using the following strategies:

- Information and Preparation: Arm yourself with knowledge about dementia. Understanding what to expect can demystify the condition and reduce fear of the unknown.
- Mindfulness and Relaxation: Techniques such as deep breathing, meditation, or yoga can help calm the mind and reduce stress. Even a few minutes a day can make a difference.

- Setting Small Goals: Focus on what can be accomplished today or this week rather than worrying about the distant future. Achieving these goals can provide a sense of control and reduce anxiety.
- Support Networks: Lean on your support network for comfort and advice. Sharing your worries with others who understand can alleviate the sense of carrying the burden alone.

Emotional Self-Care

Emotional self-care is not a luxury but a necessity for caregivers. It's about ensuring you're mentally and emotionally equipped to continue providing care. Self-care activities are meant to help you heal, put your mind at ease, and lift the weight off your shoulders. These can be wide-ranged, depending on what makes you feel better. However, there are a few standard practices that you can try:

- Time for Yourself: Set aside time for activities that recharge your emotional batteries. Whether it's a hobby, exercise, or quiet time to read or soak in a bath, these moments can help sustain your emotional well-being.
- Journaling: Writing about your experiences, thoughts, and feelings can be a therapeutic way to process emotions. It can also remind you of the challenges you've faced and overcome.
- Support from Peers or Professionals: Sometimes, talking to someone who's been in your shoes or a professional who understands can offer the validation and strategies you need to cope. Don't hesitate to reach out for help.
- Celebrating the Positives: Amidst the challenges, there are moments of joy, love, and connection. Acknowledge and celebrate these, letting them remind you of the value and impact of your care.

Caring for someone with dementia is an emotional whirlwind, marked by moments of joy, sadness, guilt, and worry. Navigating this landscape requires compassion, not just for your loved one, but for yourself. Through strategies for managing guilt, grief, and anxiety and prioritizing emotional self-care, you can find a balance that allows you to provide care while maintaining your emotional health. Remember, taking care of yourself isn't just about your well-being; it's about being in the best position to care for your loved one.

Self-Care: Strategies to Avoid Burnout

Burnout creeps silently into the lives of caregivers, a gradual accumulation of stress, fatigue, and emotional weariness. It's the consequence of days, weeks, and months spent prioritizing the needs of a loved one with dementia above one's own. Recognizing the early warning signs is pivotal. These signs might manifest as a constant feeling of tiredness, irritability, or detachment from the person you're caring for. You might notice sleep disturbances, changes in appetite, or a lack of interest in activities that once brought joy. Consider these temporary setbacks and indicators that it's time to reinforce your self-care practices.

Thankfully, with enough research and experience, we know what can help caregivers under these challenging circumstances. This section will cover the strategies you can employ to regain your inner strength.

Practical Self-Care

Self-care encompasses many activities and practices that restore energy, reduce stress, and promote well-being. Consider integrating these into your routine:

- Daily Movement: Regular physical activity, whether yoga, walking, or dancing, can significantly boost your mood and energy levels. It doesn't have to be time-consuming; even short, 10-minute sessions can make a difference.
- Hobbies and Interests: Reconnect with activities that bring you happiness. Whether painting, gardening, or playing an instrument, these pursuits provide a necessary escape and a sense of normalcy.

- Mindfulness and Meditation: Mindfulness practices can help center your thoughts and reduce stress. If you are unaware of where to start, then apps offering guided meditations can be a convenient way to start. You can also watch guided meditations on YouTube.
- Relaxation Techniques: Techniques such as deep breathing, progressive muscle relaxation, or a warm bath can help soothe the mind and body, preparing you for a better night's sleep.

Asking for Help

One of the toughest hurdles for caregivers is acknowledging when they need help and then asking for it. Remember, seeking assistance is a sign of strength, not weakness. Here's how you can approach it:

- Identify Specific Needs: Before reaching out, pinpoint what kind of help you need. Is it someone to watch your loved one while you take a break? Assistance with household chores? Identifying specific tasks makes it easier for others to provide support.
- Use a Direct Approach: Be clear and direct when asking for help. People are often willing to assist but may not know how. By stating your needs explicitly, you allow them to step in effectively.
- Explore Professional Services: Consider professional services for tasks requiring specialized skills or respite care. Home health aides, adult day care centers, or professional caregivers can give you the break you need.
- Leverage Online Platforms: Platforms like social media groups or caregiver forums can be excellent resources for finding support, sharing responsibilities, or simply connecting with others who understand your situation.

Maintaining Personal Health

Neglecting your health can diminish your ability to provide care. Ensuring you prioritize self-care is essential to prevent burnout and maintain the strength and resilience needed to provide adequate care for your loved one.

To avoid this pitfall, prioritize your health by:

- Regular Health Check-ups: Stay on top of your health by keeping routine medical appointments. These check-ups can catch potential health issues early or provide reassurance about your well-being.
- Nutritious Eating: A balanced diet fuels the body and mind. Try to incorporate a variety of fruits, vegetables, lean proteins, and whole grains into your meals. Planning and preparing healthy snacks can make it easier to eat well, even on busy days.
- Quality Sleep: Good sleep is foundational to coping with stress and preventing burnout. Establish a regular sleep schedule, create a restful environment, and avoid caffeine and screens before bedtime to improve sleep quality.
- Hydration: Drinking enough water is often overlooked but is crucial for maintaining energy levels and overall health. Keep a water bottle handy as a reminder to stay hydrated throughout the day.

In recognizing the signs of burnout and implementing strategies for self-care, you safeguard not only your well-being but also your capacity to provide compassionate, effective care for your loved one with dementia. It's a delicate balance that requires attention and adjustment as circumstances change. But by prioritizing self-care, you ensure that you can continue to be a source of strength, support, and love for your loved one.

Finding Strength in Support Systems

The social and emotional challenges of dementia caregiving can often feel isolating and overwhelming. But you don't have to deal with everything alone. Even if you have been taking care of a loved one with dementia for years, you can still go out and build support networks for yourself. You may learn great new lessons from others and never feel alone again. In dementia caregiving, forging connections and harnessing the strength of community resources can transform the caregiving experience from isolation to support and shared wisdom.

This section offers guidance on cultivating a robust support network, tapping into local services, navigating online platforms, and engaging in advocacy efforts. Each of these avenues opens doors to resources, advice, and companionship that can lighten the load of caregiving responsibilities.

Building a Support Network

Creating a support network involves reaching out and connecting with those who understand the nuances of dementia caregiving. This network can include:

- Family and Friends: Start by engaging family members and friends in open conversations about the caregiving needs and how they can contribute. Even small acts of support can provide significant relief.
- Caregiving Communities: Local caregiving groups offer a platform to meet others in similar situations. The camaraderie found in these groups can be a source of comfort and practical advice.
- Healthcare Professionals: Establishing a rapport with your loved one's healthcare providers ensures you have access to medical advice and insights into managing dementia symptoms effectively.

- Volunteers: Many communities have volunteers willing to lend a hand, whether providing companionship to your loved one or assisting with errands. Local volunteer organizations or faith-based groups are good places to start.

Each strand of this network brings unique forms of support and weaves a safety net that promises resilience and companionship for caregivers and those they care for.

Leveraging Local Resources

The community surrounding you is a reservoir of resources that can alleviate many of the challenges associated with dementia caregiving. Exploring these resources brings practical benefits and deepens your connection to the broader community, reminding you that you're not navigating this path alone. Here are a few that you can consider:

- Respite Care Services: These services offer temporary care for your loved one, allowing you much-needed breaks. Explore options through local elder care agencies or community centers.
- Support Groups: Regular meetings with local support groups provide a space to share experiences and strategies, reducing feelings of isolation.
- Dementia Care Services: Local health departments often have lists of specialized services for those with dementia, including daycare programs, home health aides, and therapeutic activities.
- Educational Workshops: Workshops and seminars on dementia care can equip you with new skills and knowledge, empowering you to tackle caregiving challenges confidently.

Online Communities and Resources

The digital realm offers a vast support network accessible right from your home. These online platforms can be particularly valuable for those who may find it challenging to attend in-person meetings due to caregiving responsibilities or geographic constraints.

- Forums and Social Media Groups: Platforms like Facebook, Reddit, and specialized caregiving websites host groups where caregivers can ask questions, share advice, or vent in a supportive environment.
- Educational Websites: Websites dedicated to dementia care, such as the Alzheimer's Association or Mayo Clinic, provide information on symptoms, care strategies, legal considerations, and more.
- Webinars and Online Courses: Many organizations offer free or low-cost webinars and courses on caregiving topics, allowing you to learn from experts and experienced caregivers.
- Virtual Support Meetings: Video conferencing tools have made it possible to join support group meetings from anywhere, offering flexibility to those whose schedules or locations would otherwise limit their participation.

Engaging with these online resources allows you to tap into a global support community, ensuring you can access help and information whenever needed.

Advocacy and Assistance

Becoming an advocate for dementia care helps shape better policies and services and provides a sense of purpose and empowerment. You become the voice of your loved one and all those suffering from a similar condition, advocating for understanding and empathy from society. You can focus on many aspects as an advocate, each calling for alleviating a substantial subset of problems.

- Policy Advocacy: Contact your local and national representatives to advocate for policies that support dementia caregivers and those in their care. This can include funding for dementia care services, support for caregiver health and well-being, and research into dementia treatments.

- Community Education: Offer to share your caregiving experiences and insights through community talks or articles for local newspapers or newsletters. Educating the public about dementia can foster greater understanding and support within the community.
- Fundraising and Volunteering: Participate in or organize fundraising events for dementia research or local services. Volunteering your time for dementia-related causes can also make a significant impact.
- Connecting with Advocacy Groups: Join existing advocacy groups working on dementia care issues. These groups often have established platforms and resources that can amplify your efforts.

Through advocacy, you not only contribute to the betterment of dementia care but also find a sense of solidarity and shared purpose with fellow caregivers and advocates. It's a powerful way to make a difference, extending the impact of your caregiving journey beyond your immediate circle.

Planning and Resources for Dementia Care

Let's be honest: if there is one thing that essentially governs the quality of life we can afford ourselves and extend to those we care for, it is money. Managing finances is a significant part of caregiving, regardless of whether the patient is suffering. And another honest bit is that caregiving is expensive and can be debilitating for someone without savings. This makes it crucial for caregivers to learn caregiving's long-term and short-term costs and how they must budget and plan their resources to meet their needs. Caring for a loved one with dementia brings significant expenses, ranging from medical treatments to necessary modifications in living spaces. Here, we explore managing these costs effectively, ensuring your loved one receives the best care possible without compromising your financial health.

Understanding the Costs

Dementia care encompasses a broad spectrum of expenses that can accumulate over time. These include but are not limited to:

- Medical Treatments: Regular consultations, medications, and therapies contribute to ongoing healthcare expenses.
- Home Care: Hiring caregivers or enrolling in adult day care services ensures your loved one's needs are met when you're not available.
- Living Modifications: Making your home safer and more accessible, such as installing grab bars or ramps, requires an upfront investment.
- Specialized Equipment: Items like medical alert systems or cognitive therapy tools can enhance safety and quality of life.

Acknowledging these costs early on allows for better planning and management, mitigating the risk of financial strain down the line.

Financial Planning

Creating a solid financial plan is critical in managing the costs of dementia care. This plan should include:

- Budgeting: Develop a detailed budget for all caregiving expenses, ensuring you clearly understand your finances.
- Savings and Investments: Consider setting aside funds specifically for long-term care needs. Investing in products that offer growth can help offset future costs.
- Insurance: Review existing insurance policies (health, long-term care, life) to understand what aspects of dementia care are covered and to what extent.
- Exploring Benefits and Aids: Many organizations offer financial assistance for dementia care. Identifying these resources can provide much-needed relief.

Taking these steps secures the necessary funds for quality care and protects your financial future, so you're not vulnerable due to caregiving costs.

Government and Private Assistance

Various programs and foundations offer financial support for those caring for someone with dementia. These include:

- Medicare and Medicaid: While Medicare coverage is limited, it can cover certain aspects of dementia care. Medicaid, on the other hand, might offer more extensive benefits for those who qualify.
- Veterans Benefits: Veterans and their spouses may be eligible for benefits that can help cover the costs of dementia care.
- Non-Profit Organizations: Many non-profits provide grants, subsidies, or services at reduced costs for families affected by dementia.
- Community Programs: Local government and community organizations often have programs to assist with healthcare, home modifications, or respite care.

Thorough research into these options can uncover valuable resources, reducing the financial burden of dementia care.

Legal Planning

For caregivers tasked with ensuring the well-being of their loved ones, understanding the legal aspects of financial planning is not just advisable; it's imperative. Taking necessary legal steps secures your loved one's economic legacy. It provides peace of mind, knowing their wishes will be respected and their assets utilized as intended. These legal duties may include:

- Wills and Trusts: Establishing a will or trust helps protect assets and ensures your loved one's wishes are honored.

- Power of Attorney: Assigning someone the power of attorney for financial decisions can safeguard against mismanagement as dementia progresses.
- Living Will: A living will outline your loved one's wishes regarding medical treatment, providing clear guidance during difficult times.
- Estate Planning: Consulting with a legal expert in estate planning can help maximize asset protection and minimize taxes, preserving more funds for care.

As we wrap up this exploration of the financial side of dementia care, it's clear that it requires careful planning, research, and a proactive approach. From understanding the costs involved to leveraging government and private resources, each step moves toward securing quality care for your loved one without compromising your financial well-being. Additionally, legal planning is pivotal in safeguarding assets and ensuring wishes are honored. While the path may seem daunting, know that you're not alone. Resources and support are available; seek them online or in your local dementia care centers. Remember to stay in touch with your support networks and work to make things easier for yourself; you deserve it.

As we move to the next chapter, remember that financial planning is just one piece of the puzzle. The emotional, physical, and logistical challenges of caregiving also demand attention and resources. The following chapters will address these aspects more deeply, offering strategies and insights to support you and your loved one through this journey. By this time, I hope you are taking notes or journaling the tips that fill the gaps in your caregiving methods. Journaling will help you stay abreast of what you are learning and help you share it forward as you advocate for the cause or help another fellow caregiver out in your support network. You've got this.

CHAPTER 3

CRAFTING CONNECTIONS

The most fatal thing a man can do is try to stand alone. The closest thing to being cared for is to care for someone else. – Carson McCullers.

I magine sitting down with a puzzle, pieces scattered across the table. Some pieces fit perfectly, while others don't seem to belong anywhere. Communicating with someone living with dementia can feel a lot like solving this puzzle. It's about finding the right pieces —words, gestures, tones—that click into place, creating moments of understanding and connection. In this chapter, I will share the nuances of effectively communicating with those experiencing dementia, emphasizing techniques that foster meaningful interactions.

Adapting Your Perspective

Life for someone with dementia is drastically different; their feelings, emotions, and perceptions are not always grounded in the reality around them. It's almost as if they are on a different plane of existence. This makes it even more crucial for caregivers to build an environment where their perspectives and emotions hold equal regard.

To truly reach someone with dementia, stepping into their reality is crucial. It's about understanding the world from their viewpoint, which may differ vastly from yours. This shift in perspective is not about agreeing or disagreeing with their perceptions but acknowledging their experiences as valid. For instance, if they mention seeing a childhood friend who has long passed away, instead of correcting them, engage in a conversation about that friend. This approach maintains dignity and fosters a sense of safety and understanding. There are many ways to promote this level of care and communication, and I will share a few in the following section.

Simplifying Language

The way we frame our words can make a world of difference. Language is a high function of our brains, complex and multilayered. Our brains form words after thinking and processing received and stored information. Using language enables us to engage in metacognition, the process of thinking about our thinking. It is a deeper state of self-awareness. However, as dementia is a neurodegenerative syndrome, it significantly diminishes human ability to process and produce language. Understanding this is at the core of communication and dementia care. So here are some strategies to simplify language effectively:

- Use short, clear sentences, focusing on one idea at a time. Instead of saying, "Could you possibly get dressed before breakfast so we're not rushing to make it to your appointment on time?" try, "Let's get dressed for breakfast."
- Choose direct questions or statements that require simple or yes/no responses. Ask, "Do you want tea?" instead of, "What would you like to drink?"
- Avoid idioms, sarcasm, or complex vocabulary that might

confuse you. Stick to literal language that conveys precisely what you mean.

Non-Verbal Communication

Words are just one piece of the puzzle. Non-verbal cues often speak louder, especially when verbal communication becomes challenging. Consider these points:

- Maintain eye contact to convey your attention and care.
- Use touch to provide reassurance. A gentle hand on the shoulder can be comforting.
- Pay attention to your tone of voice. A calm, warm tone can soothe anxieties and convey your message more effectively than words alone.
- Watch for their non-verbal cues, too. Body language, facial expressions, and even changes in breathing can provide insights into their feelings and needs.

Patience and Repetition

Patience truly is a virtue in dementia care. So here are a few things to understand:

- It may take time for your loved one to process information and respond. Please give them the space to do so without rushing.
- Repetition might be necessary, but repeating information or questions calmly and reassuringly is important. If they don't grasp something the first time, try rephrasing it or using different words.
- Recognize that some days will be better than others. Flexibility and patience are crucial to adapting to the fluctuating nature of dementia.

Real-life Strategies

You will find communication barriers at every turn in dementia care. Therefore, preparing yourself for real-life situations is advisable so that you are not anxious when faced with communication challenges. Here are a few examples of real-life situations and strategies to overcome communication barriers in dementia care:

- During Meals: Simplify choices by visually presenting two options rather than open-endedly asking what they'd like to eat. This makes deciding easier for them and can prevent feelings of overwhelm.
- In Social Settings: Before a family gathering, gently remind your loved one who each person is and what their relationship is. Use photos if helpful, and encourage family members to approach calmly, introducing themselves even if they're familiar.
- When Experiencing Confusion: If they become disoriented or upset about not recognizing their surroundings, validate their feelings instead of insisting they're at home. Use calming non-verbal cues and gently guide the conversation to a comforting topic or activity.

Incorporating these communication strategies into daily interactions can transform moments of frustration into opportunities for connection and understanding. Remember, each person with dementia is unique, and what works for one may not work for another. It's about trying different approaches, observing what resonates, and always leading with empathy and respect.

Tools and Resources

Here are some practical tools to support caregivers in applying these communication techniques. These tools and resources are necessary because they can help improve communication with individuals with dementia, reducing frustration and enhancing overall caregiving experiences.

- Checklist for Simplified Communication: A handy guide to ensure your verbal and non-verbal communication is clear and comforting.
- Reflection Journal: Keeping a journal can be a valuable tool for noting what communication strategies work well and which don't, helping you tailor your approach over time.
- Online Courses and Workshops: Many organizations offer training geared towards improving communication with individuals living with dementia. These can be invaluable resources for developing your skills.

It would be best to acknowledge that communication in dementia care is both an art and a science. It requires understanding, patience, and creativity to find the right combination of words, tones, and gestures that reach through the fog of confusion. By adapting your perspective, simplifying language, leveraging non-verbal cues, and embracing patience; you create a bridge to your loved one's world. Through these connections, we find moments of joy, understanding, and deep human connection, reminding us of the power of communication in navigating the challenges of dementia care.

The Art of Listening: Responding to Unspoken Needs

Creating a safe environment and a strong bond with fellow humans means being there for them whenever needed. And most of the time, being there requires lending a sincere ear for them to express themselves. This need to be understood remains with us, regardless of our life stage or circumstances. Similarly, listening in dementia care transcends the act of hearing. It's an engagement of the heart, a deliberate tuning-in to the emotions, fears, and needs often unnoticed. This section explores the nuances of listening deeply to someone with dementia, offering insights into how caregivers can respond compassionately to spoken and unspoken messages.

Active Listening Skills

Active listening is the cornerstone of effective communication, especially when interacting with individuals experiencing dementia. It involves fully concentrating on what is being said rather than passively 'hearing' the speaker's message. Here are techniques that underline empathy and validation:

- Mirroring Emotions: This technique involves reflecting the emotions you perceive in the speaker. If your loved one expresses frustration, acknowledge that frustration by saying, "You seem upset about this," which shows understanding and acceptance.
- Acknowledging Feelings: Sometimes, an individual seeks validation of their feelings. Simple statements like, "That sounds hard," can go a long way in making them feel heard and supported.
- Follow-up Questions: Asking questions based on what the person has just shared demonstrates genuine interest and encourages them to share more. It can be as simple as, "Can you tell me more about that?"
- Summarizing and Repeating Back: Occasionally rephrase what your loved one has said and repeat it to them. This ensures you've understood correctly and makes them feel valued and listened to.

Recognizing Non-Verbal Cues

Much of our communication is non-verbal, conveyed through body language, facial expressions, and even silence. For someone with dementia, these cues can be especially significant. Recognizing and responding to them requires attentiveness and sensitivity. These cues can be different for different people. As you know your loved one best, you should be able to read between the lines and recognize unsaid emotions. Here are a few things to be attentive to:

- Facial Expressions: A furrowed brow or a smile can convey volumes about how the person is feeling. Respond to these expressions by commenting on them or adjusting your approach accordingly.
- Body Language: Notice if they lean forward when engaged or pull away when uncomfortable. These cues can guide how you continue the conversation or activity.
- Physical Movements: Agitation might be expressed through pacing or hand-wringing. Calmness might be seen in relaxed shoulders and a steady gaze. Respond to these signals with appropriate interventions, such as a calming activity or a change of environment.

Creating a Safe Space for Expression

For individuals with dementia, expressing themselves can be daunting, primarily if their communication abilities have been affected. Therefore, it is vital to create an environment where they feel safe and encouraged to express themselves. Here's what you can do:

- Maintain a Calm Environment: Reduce background noise and distractions that can cause confusion or overwhelm. A quiet, peaceful setting encourages focus and makes it easier for your loved ones to express themselves.
- Be Present: Give them your full attention, showing that what they say is important. Avoid multitasking during conversations.
- Use Encouraging Body Language: Open, welcoming body language—like uncrossed arms and a gentle nod—encourages people to share their thoughts and feelings.
- Respect Their Pace: Allow them to speak without rushing them. If they struggle to find words, resist the urge to finish sentences for them unless they seek help.

Encouraging Expression

Finding alternate ways for your loved one to express themselves can be rewarding. Music, art, and photographs are powerful tools for unlocking memories and enabling communication:

- Music: Play songs from their youth or other significant periods in their life. Music can evoke memories and feelings, sparking conversations or simply bringing joy.
- Art: Engage in simple art projects that allow for creative expression without the pressure of finding the right words. Painting or drawing can be therapeutic and a source of connection.
- Photographs: Use photo albums to encourage reminiscing. Ask open-ended questions about the pictures to invite stories and memories.

These activities provide avenues for expression and enrich the lives of individuals with dementia, offering joy and a sense of accomplishment. Through active listening, recognizing non-verbal cues, creating safe spaces for expression, and encouraging alternative forms of communication, caregivers can foster deeper connections with their loved ones. In these moments of shared understanding and empathy, the true essence of caregiving is revealed.

Handling Agitation: De-escalation Strategies That Work

Caring for someone with dementia often means encountering moments of agitation. These instances can be as perplexing as they are stressful, both for the caregiver and the person experiencing them. Dementia patients may experience agitation due to various factors. These may include physical discomfort, unmet needs, confusion, frustration, or environmental changes. Sometimes, it may also not be possible to figure out the cause of their agitation. In all these cases, caregivers must remain calm and patient while seeking professional assistance and guidance to manage and address the agitation.

Understanding how to manage these situations effectively is crucial, not only for the well-being of the individual with dementia but also for maintaining a peaceful and nurturing care environment.

Identifying Triggers

The first step in managing agitation is pinpointing what sparks it. Common triggers include environmental factors like noise or poor lighting, physical discomfort, and emotional distress. Sometimes, even a break in routine can lead to unease. Here are strategies for identifying and mitigating these triggers:

- Keep a Diary: Note instances of agitation, including the time, setting, and possible causes. Over time, patterns may emerge, offering clues to specific triggers.
- Review Basic Needs: Ensure basic needs are met. Hunger, thirst, or the need for a restroom can cause distress. Regularly check for these needs as a preventative measure.
- Minimize Stressors: Pay attention to the environment. Is it too loud, too bright, or too cluttered? Adjusting these elements can help reduce potential triggers.

By becoming adept at recognizing what precedes episodes of agitation, you can take proactive steps to minimize these triggers, creating a more comfortable environment for your loved one.

Calming Techniques

Having a repertoire of calming techniques can help soothe tension when agitation arises. Everyone is unique, so what works for one might not work for another. Experiment with these strategies to find the most effective approach:

- Redirection: Gently shift focus to a different, more calming activity. This could be looking through a photo album,

listening to a favorite piece of music, or stepping outside for fresh air.
- Find a Quiet Environment: If the surroundings contribute to the agitation, moving to a quieter, less stimulating space can help.
- Use Calming Music or Activities: Soft, soothing music or engaging in a simple, enjoyable activity like folding laundry or coloring can have a calming effect.
- Deep Breathing: Guiding your loved one through deep breathing exercises can help reduce tension. Demonstrate by doing it together, emphasizing slow, deep breaths.

These techniques help manage immediate episodes of agitation and contribute to a more serene daily life for you and your loved one.

Dementia-friendly Environment

The environment plays a significant role in the well-being of someone with dementia. An area that is too stimulating or unfamiliar can quickly become overwhelming, leading to agitation. Creating a dementia-friendly space involves:

- Reduce Noise: Keep the environment as quiet as possible. Background noise from a television or radio might be distracting, so consider turning them off or down.
- Ensure Adequate Lighting: Poor lighting can cause confusion and fear. Make sure rooms are well-lit, using natural light where possible.
- Create Safe Spaces: Arrange furniture and remove clutter to create clear pathways. This helps prevent falls and reduces anxiety about navigating the space.
- Personalize the Room: Having familiar items can make the space feel safe and recognizable. Family photos, favorite books, or a cherished blanket can provide comfort and security.

By thoughtfully arranging the living environment, you can prevent many situations that might lead to agitation, fostering a sense of calm and safety.

When to Seek Professional Help

While many instances of agitation can be managed with the strategies mentioned, there are times when professional help is necessary. Recognizing the signs that more specialized care is needed is crucial. Here are indications that it might be time to seek outside assistance:

- Persistent Agitation: If episodes of agitation become frequent or intense, despite attempts at de-escalation, it might indicate an underlying issue that requires professional evaluation.
- Physical Aggression: If agitation escalates to physical aggression, it's essential to seek help to ensure the safety of both the caregiver and the person with dementia.
- Change in Health Status: Sudden changes in behavior or well-being could signal a health issue that needs medical attention.
- Caregiver Stress: Professional support can offer relief and guidance if managing agitation significantly impacts your health and well-being.

Reaching out for help can involve consulting with a healthcare provider familiar with dementia care, seeking advice from a dementia support organization, or considering the services of a professional caregiver trained in managing behavioral symptoms of dementia. Remember, asking for assistance is not a sign of failure but an important step in providing the best possible care for your loved one and ensuring your well-being as a caregiver.

Dementia care is complex; it will challenge you and bring moments that test your patience and resilience. Yet, with the right strategies and a deep understanding of how to manage agitation, you can create a nurturing environment that supports the well-being of your loved one.

Each step is a testament to your commitment to compassionate care, from identifying triggers to implementing calming techniques, adjusting the environment, and knowing when to seek professional help.

Innovative Tools for Communication

Thankfully, we live in a time when technology facilitates caregiving, making it manageable. It has undoubtedly evolved the communication landscape, bridging the gap between caregivers and their loved ones. The advent of various technological aids has opened up new avenues for interaction, making it possible to maintain a connection even as the disease progresses. Therefore, in this section, I will share the assortment of tools at our disposal, from speech-generating devices to apps specifically designed for those with dementia, and explore how these innovations can enhance daily communication and enrich the lives of caregivers and their loved ones.

Technology Aids

The digital era brings gadgets and applications meticulously crafted to ease communication challenges. Speech-generating devices, for instance, have been a revelation, empowering individuals who struggle with verbal expression to convey their thoughts and needs with the touch of a button. These devices range from simple picture-based apps to more sophisticated systems synthesizing speech from typed text. Additionally, numerous apps cater to the specific needs of dementia patients and their caregivers, offering features like medication reminders, activity scheduling, and even virtual companionship through chatbots designed to engage users in conversation. Such tools not only facilitate smoother daily interactions but also offer a semblance of independence to those living with dementia.

Visual Aids

Visual aids serve as another effective tool in facilitating communication and daily activities. Picture boards, for example, can help make choices clearer for someone with dementia. Visual cues can simplify the decision-making process, Whether deciding what to wear or selecting a meal. Digital photo frames with family pictures and short videos can also prompt conversations and encourage reminiscing. Moreover, apps that allow for the customization of visual aids—enabling caregivers to upload familiar faces, objects, and places—can be particularly helpful in creating a comforting and recognizable environment for individuals with dementia.

Educational Resources

The quest for knowledge on effectively communicating with their loved ones is ongoing for caregivers. The digital world is abundant with resources that cater to this need. Online platforms offer courses, webinars, and interactive workshops that cover a broad spectrum of topics, from understanding dementia-related communication challenges to learning specific strategies for enhancing interaction. These resources equip caregivers with the necessary skills and provide a community of support, sharing, and learning, ensuring they never feel they are navigating this path alone.

Personalized Playlists

Music holds a unique power to unlock memories and elicit emotions, making personalized playlists an invaluable tool in dementia care. Compiling a selection of meaningful songs for your loved one can spark reminiscences of happy times, soothe anxiety, and even stimulate conversation. Music streaming services and apps dedicated to creating personalized playlists make this process easier, allowing caregivers to set up playlists that can be easily accessed anytime. Whether it's the tunes they danced to in their youth or the melodies they hummed to their children, these personalized compilations can be a source of comfort and joy. Remember, anything that your loved one may enjoy, it may be any other art form, can be used to build a deeper connection and have conversations with your loved ones.

By now, you are aware of multiple techniques and strategies for building a deeper connection with your loved one with dementia. You may have been practicing some of these methods already, a testament to your great caregiving. Just as important as it is to build a connection with your loved one, it is also crucial for you to believe in yourself and your ability to take care of them. Communication is a two-way street; not only does it benefit the individual with dementia, but it also reassures you that you are providing quality care.

As we wrap up this exploration of technological innovations in dementia care, we're reminded of the power of connection. Despite the obstacles dementia presents, our ability to reach out, understand, and engage with our loved ones remains undiminished. We reaffirm our commitment to their dignity, history, and enduring bond with every tool we employ. As we move forward, let's carry the lessons learned here, ready to apply them in our journey ahead, always looking for new ways to enhance the lives of those we care for.

CHAPTER 4

ANCHORING THE DAY

"One person caring about another represents life's greatest value."
- Jim Rohn.

Picture yourself embarking on a hiking journey through a dense forest without a trail guide. The forest, with its towering trees and winding paths, presents a myriad of unknowns. Similarly, navigating life with dementia can often feel like trekking through unfamiliar terrain without a guidebook. Developing a daily care plan serves as our trail guide, offering insight and guidance amid the unpredictable twists and turns of dementia care. It's not about adhering strictly to predefined paths or routines but rather about establishing waypoints that offer direction while adapting to the ever-changing landscape of caregiving challenges and victories.

Routine Matters: Establishing a Daily Care Plan

A consistent daily routine offers many benefits for individuals with dementia and their caregivers. It reduces confusion by creating a predictable environment, thereby enhancing feelings of security and comfort. For the caregiver, a routine can significantly decrease day-to-day decision fatigue, allowing more energy to be focused on meaningful interactions and care.

- Morning Calmness: Starting the day with a calming activity, like listening to soft music or enjoying a cup of tea, can set a positive tone for the rest of the day.
- Mealtime Regularity: Having meals at the same time every day helps regulate the body's internal clock, contributing to better digestion and overall well-being.
- Evening Wind-down: Establishing a soothing evening routine, such as reading a book or a gentle hand massage with lotion, can aid in better sleep for the individual and the caregiver.

Creating a Flexible Schedule

Flexibility is vital in a dementia care plan due to the condition's unpredictable nature. It allows caregivers to adapt to changing needs, tailor care to individual preferences, cope with new challenges, and promote dignity and independence. By remaining flexible, caregivers can provide more effective support and enhance the quality of life for individuals with dementia and themselves. Here's how to balance structure with the need for adaptability in your care plan:

- Prioritize: Identify the most critical activities and routines that need consistency, like medication times and meals, and build flexibility around these pillars.
- Plan for Downtime: Incorporate rest periods and unstructured time to accommodate fluctuating energy levels and mood.
- Adjust as Needed: Be prepared to modify the day's plan based

on how your loved one is feeling. Some days might allow for more activities, while others require a slower pace.

Involving the Individual

Involvement in the care plan fosters a sense of agency and respect. Tailoring participation to the individual's abilities and preferences can enhance their cooperation and satisfaction with daily routines.

- Choice: Offer choices within the routine, such as between two outfit options or activities. This supports autonomy and decision-making skills.
- Participation: Encourage participation in manageable tasks, like setting the table, which can boost confidence and provide a sense of purpose.
- Feedback: Pay attention to nonverbal cues that indicate preferences, adjusting the plan to align more closely with the individual's comfort and enjoyment.

Documentation and Communication

A well-documented routine ensures consistent care, especially when multiple caregivers are involved.

- Care Plan Folder: Keep a folder with the daily routine, medication schedule, and other pertinent information. This serves as a quick reference for all caregivers.
- Digital Tools: Utilize apps or digital calendars that can be shared among family members and caregivers for real-time updates and coordination.
- Regular Check-ins: Meet with family members and other caregivers to discuss the care plan, share observations, and make necessary adjustments.

Incorporating visuals can significantly aid in the communication and execution of the daily care plan. Consider creating a visual daily

schedule, using symbols or pictures for each activity. This not only helps the individual with dementia understand the day's structure but also offers caregivers a clear, at-a-glance overview of the day's plan.

Crafting a care plan for someone with dementia is like drawing a map in the sand; it provides direction but acknowledges the unpredictability of dementia care. A routine offers the structure needed to navigate daily challenges, while flexibility allows for the individuality and changing needs of the person at the heart of care. By involving the individual in their care plan, documenting, and communicating effectively, caregivers can create a day filled with moments of connection, understanding, and joy amidst the unpredictabilities of dementia care.

Creative Engagement for Mind and Soul

Engaging individuals with dementia in activities that resonate with their personal history, interests, and current capabilities can significantly enhance their quality of life. It honors their past and celebrates their present. Each activity—through tailored tasks, sensory experiences, cognitive exercises, or outdoor explorations—adds color, texture, and depth, enriching their daily lives with moments of joy, achievement, and connection.

Tailored Activities

Selecting activities that echo an individual's history and passions ensures these pursuits are enjoyable and deeply meaningful. Here's how to craft these personalized experiences:

- Life Story Exploration: Use their life story as a guide. A former gardener might enjoy tending to house plants or arranging floral bouquets, while a retired teacher could enjoy reading to children at a local library.
- Adapting to Abilities: Modify activities to match their current skill level. For instance, someone who loved baking might now

enjoy assisting with more straightforward tasks like stirring batter or decorating cookies.

- Interactive Reminiscence: Incorporate elements from their past into activities. Playing their favorite music from when they were young or recreating a meal from a significant event can spark memories and conversations.

Sensory Stimulation

Sensory activities tap into the basic senses—sight, sound, touch, taste, and smell—to evoke responses and engage individuals at a fundamental level. They bypass cognitive impairments and tap into primal sensory experiences. These activities stimulate memories, emotions, and connections, reducing agitation and promoting relaxation. Here are a few ways to incorporate sensory stimulation:

- Tactile Mats and Objects: Craft mats with various textures or provide objects like worry beads, soft fabrics, or textured balls to explore by touch.
- Aromatherapy: Use scented lotions during massage or diffuse essential oils like lavender or peppermint to create a calming or stimulating environment.
- Taste Testing: Organize a taste-testing session with different flavors of jelly, fruit, or small bites of various dishes, encouraging them to describe what they taste.
- Soundscapes: Play sounds of nature, such as birdsong or rain, or use instruments like rain sticks or chimes to provide auditory stimulation.

Cognitive Exercises

Along with fun activities, cognitive exercises are also necessary to enhance brain function. Cognitive activities stimulate the brain, potentially slowing down the progression of dementia symptoms and providing a sense of achievement. Here are some exercises that can be both fun and beneficial:

- Puzzle Solving: Offer puzzles with large, easy-to-handle pieces or simple crosswords and word searches that align with their ability level.
- Memory Boxes: Create a 'memory box' filled with items related to a particular theme or period of their life. Going through the box can stimulate discussions and reminiscence.
- Sorting and Organizing: Engage them in sorting objects by color, size, or category. This can be as simple as organizing buttons, coins, or cards.
- Storytelling with Props: Use photographs, postcards, or objects as prompts to tell stories or describe memories. This can be a shared activity that enhances connection.

Outdoor Activities

The great outdoors offers many opportunities for physical activity, connection with nature, and sensory stimulation. Here's how to safely enjoy the benefits of being outside:

- Nature Walks: Short walks in safe, familiar areas can offer fresh air and a change of scenery. Tailor the length and difficulty of the walk to their comfort and energy levels.
- Gardening: Simple gardening activities, such as watering plants, weeding, or potting flowers, provide a sense of accomplishment and connection to the cycle of life.
- Bird Watching: Set up a bird feeder visible from a window or sit outside in a quiet spot to observe birds. Identifying different species can be an engaging activity.
- Picnics: Having a meal outdoors, in a park, or even in the backyard can be a delightful change of pace. Ensure comfort with accessible seating and shade.

Incorporating these diverse activities into the caregiving routine offers individuals with dementia opportunities to engage with the world around them in meaningful ways. From tailored tasks that echo their interests and history to sensory experiences that awaken the senses, cognitive exercises that challenge the mind, and outdoor explorations that reconnect them with nature, each activity is a step toward enriching their daily experiences. By carefully selecting and adapting these pursuits, caregivers can ensure that their loved ones continue to enjoy a high quality of life filled with moments of joy, achievement, and connection.

Behavioral Insights into Challenging Behaviors

Imagine sitting with your loved one who has dementia in a cozy living room one afternoon. As you engage in conversation, you notice them becoming increasingly restless, fidgeting with their hands and pacing around the room. Instead of feeling overwhelmed, you take a moment to observe closely. Soon, you realize that their agitation is a sign of discomfort. So, with a gentle touch and reassuring words, you guide them to a more comfortable position, and gradually, their restlessness subsides. In this imaginary scenario, you recognize the importance of interpreting sudden behavioral changes as forms of communication, offering valuable insights into their unspoken needs and emotions.

You may have come across such behaviors in your caregiving journey. The behaviors that may arise are varied, often unexpected, and can be a source of stress and confusion for both the caregiver and the individual. It's crucial, then, to approach these behaviors not as obstacles but as windows into the unspoken needs and emotions of our loved ones.

Understanding the Cause

No matter how perplexing it may seem, each behavior has an underlying reason. It could be an attempt to communicate a need, an expression of discomfort, or a response to an overwhelming situation. For instance, a sudden outburst could be the result of physical pain, while repeated questions may stem from anxiety or confusion about their environment. Recognizing these behaviors as forms of communication requires us to become detectives, piecing together clues to understand the needs our loved ones cannot articulate.

- Observation: Pay close attention to when and where these behaviors occur. Is there a pattern or a trigger that seems to initiate them?
- Environment Assessment: Consider whether something in their surroundings could contribute to their distress. Noise, clutter, or even the presence of unfamiliar people can be overwhelming.
- Physical Comfort: Regularly check for potential sources of discomfort. Hunger, thirst, or the need for a restroom break are basic needs that can lead to agitation if not met.

Personalized Strategies

Once the potential causes of challenging behaviors are identified, we will tailor our approach to address them effectively. This involves creativity, patience, and understanding, guided by the individual's history, preferences, and current abilities.

- Routine Adjustments: For someone who gets agitated in crowded settings, plan visits or activities during quieter times.
- Soothing Techniques: If noise is a trigger, creating a personal playlist of their favorite, calming music can provide comfort and distraction.
- Communication Adjustments: For individuals who become easily frustrated during conversations, simplify language and use visual aids or gestures to aid understanding.

Personalizing your approach not only addresses the immediate behavior but also enhances the overall well-being of your loved one, making daily interactions more enjoyable for both of you.

Professional Guidance

There are instances when behaviors become challenging to manage despite our best efforts. Seeking advice from professionals experienced in dementia care can provide new perspectives and strategies to address complex behaviors.

- Consult Healthcare Providers: A doctor can review medications and health conditions that might be influencing behavior. Sometimes, an adjustment in treatment can lead to significant improvements.
- Behavioral Therapists: Specialists in dementia care can offer behavioral modification techniques tailored to the specific needs of your loved one.
- Support Groups: Sharing experiences with other caregivers can reveal new approaches and coping strategies that have been effective in similar situations.

Leveraging professional resources broadens your toolkit for managing challenging behaviors and reinforces that you're not alone in this. There's a community of support ready to assist you.

Caring for the Caregiver

The impact of challenging behaviors on caregivers cannot be understated. The continuous cycle of managing outbursts, agitation, or resistance can lead to caregiver burnout, impacting both physical and emotional health. Recognizing the signs of stress and taking steps to care for yourself is as important as the care you provide. You always have the option to pick any activity that relaxes you. Still, if you are unsure and too exhausted to think, you may try a few of the following options:

- Self-awareness: Acknowledge your feelings of frustration, sadness, or exhaustion. Identifying these emotions is the first step in addressing them.
- Self-care Practices: Incorporating activities that promote relaxation and well-being into your daily routine can help mitigate stress. Even short breaks or a walk outside can be rejuvenating.

- Seek Support: Don't hesitate to reach out for help, whether arranging respite care to give yourself a break or talking to a counselor about the emotional toll of caregiving.

Remember, taking care of yourself isn't just beneficial for you; it directly impacts the quality of care you can provide. Prioritizing your well-being ensures you have the resilience, patience, and energy needed to navigate the challenges of dementia care with compassion and understanding. And if you feel guilty for paying attention to yourself when you are used to pouring all of your energies into your loved one's care, know that you cannot help them at all if you are not physically and mentally healthy. This reminds me of a great quote:

"Self-care is not selfish. You cannot serve from an empty vessel." – **Eleanor Brown.**

We can take away from this section that our goal isn't to suppress or control challenging behaviors but to understand and respond with empathy. By seeking to comprehend the root causes, personalizing our strategies, utilizing professional guidance, and prioritizing caregiver well-being, we create an environment where the caregiver and the individual with dementia can experience moments of joy, connection, and peace. This approach not only makes daily care more manageable but also honors the dignity and individuality of our loved ones, allowing them to navigate their world with as much comfort and understanding as possible.

Safe Spaces: Adapting Your Home for Dementia Care

Creating a home that's both welcoming and safe for a loved one with dementia involves thoughtful adjustments and a touch of creativity. It's about shaping an environment that minimizes risks while promoting independence and a sense of familiarity. Here, we'll explore practical steps to tailor your living space to the unique needs of someone navigating the changes dementia brings.

Home Safety Evaluation

Initiating a home safety evaluation is a critical first step in adapting your space. This process involves a thorough walkthrough of your home, room by room, with a keen eye for potential hazards that might not be obvious at first glance. Here's how to approach it:

- Begin with the basics: Check for loose rugs, cluttered walkways, and unstable furniture that could pose tripping hazards.
- Assess the bathroom: Consider the installation of grab bars, non-slip mats, and perhaps a shower seat to enhance safety during personal care routines.
- Kitchen safety: Evaluate the need for appliance locks and stove guards to prevent accidental burns or fires.
- Lighting: Ensure all home areas are well-lit to reduce shadows and glare, which can be confusing or disorienting.

This evaluation isn't a one-time task but an ongoing process, adapting as needs evolve.

Dementia-Friendly Design

Transforming your home into a dementia-friendly environment doesn't require a complete overhaul but targeted changes that reduce confusion and enhance navigation. Here are some suggestions:

- Clear signage: Use simple labels or pictograms to mark rooms and cabinets, making it easier for your loved one to find their way around.
- Simplify layouts: Arrange furniture in a straightforward, predictable layout, removing unnecessary items that could confuse or overwhelm.

- Color coding: Employ contrasting colors to distinguish between critical elements, like using a toilet seat in a color that stands out from the rest of the bathroom for better visibility.
- Personal touches: Fill the home with familiar objects and photos to foster a sense of comfort and belonging.

These adjustments can transform a living space into a safe harbor, anchoring your loved one in a setting that feels both manageable and welcoming.

Use of Assistive Devices

Incorporating assistive devices and home modifications can significantly bolster independence and safety. Here's a look at some valuable tools:

- Motion sensors: Install these to automatically turn lights on and off as your loved one moves through the house, reducing the risk of falls in darkened spaces.
- Door alarms: For those at risk of wandering, door alarms can alert you when exterior doors are opened, providing peace of mind.
- Communication aids: Consider devices that simplify communication, such as phones with large buttons and preset numbers for easy calling.
- Medication reminders: Automated pill dispensers can help ensure medications are taken correctly and on time, reducing the risk of missed doses.

Embracing these technologies can smooth daily routines and foster a sense of autonomy for your loved one.

Emergency Preparedness

Preparing for emergencies, including wandering or health crises, is essential to dementia care. Here's how to ensure you're ready:

- Emergency contacts: Keep a list of emergency contacts, including doctors, family members, and neighbors, in a visible and accessible place.
- Identification: Ensure your loved one carries identification or wears an ID bracelet, which is especially important for individuals prone to wandering.
- Medical information: Maintain an up-to-date record of medical conditions, medications, and care preferences, both at home and in a format that can be quickly taken to doctor's visits or hospital trips.
- Wandering plan: Develop a plan for what to do if your loved one goes missing, including who to call and where to search first.

Preparing for emergencies provides a safety net, ensuring you can respond swiftly and effectively when needed.

In tailoring your home to the needs of someone with dementia, you craft a space that's safer and more aligned with their way of experiencing the world. It's a proactive approach that acknowledges dementia's challenges while celebrating the moments of independence and joy that are still possible. From conducting a detailed safety evaluation and embracing dementia-friendly design principles to incorporating assistive devices and preparing for emergencies, each step is a stride toward creating a nurturing, secure environment where your loved one can thrive.

Nutrition and Exercise: Foundations of Physical Well-Being

Nourishing the body and engaging in physical activity are pillars for maintaining health and enhancing the quality of life for individuals with dementia. How we approach food and movement can significantly impact their well-being, mood, and cognitive function.

Dietary Considerations

Feeding the body with the proper nutrients becomes more critical as someone navigates the complexities of dementia. Changes in appetite or preference might arise, making meal times challenging. Here's how we can address these shifts:

- Balanced Diet: Focus on meals rich in fruits, vegetables, whole grains, and lean proteins. Foods high in antioxidants and omega-3 fatty acids, like berries and fish, are particularly beneficial for brain health.
- Mealtime Environment: Create a calm, distraction-free setting for meals to help focus attention on eating. A simple table setting, with contrasting colors to distinguish plates from the table, can aid in reducing confusion.
- Adapting to Preferences: Pay attention to changes in taste or food preferences. Someone who once loved spicy food may now prefer milder flavors. Experimenting with textures and flavors can help find appealing options.
- Small, Frequent Meals: If appetite decreases, smaller, nutrient-dense meals throughout the day can be more manageable than three large ones.

Hydration Strategies

Staying hydrated is crucial yet often overlooked. Dehydration can lead to confusion, irritability, and other health issues that compound the challenges of dementia. Encouraging fluid intake involves:

- Accessible Drinks: Keep a favorite cup or bottle filled with water within easy reach. Offering drinks in a clear container can help remind them to drink.
- Flavorful Options: Sometimes, plain water isn't appealing. Add fruit slices for a natural flavor boost, or offer decaffeinated herbal teas.

- Hydration Through Foods: Incorporate foods with high water content into meals. Soups, smoothies, fruits like watermelon and oranges, and vegetables like cucumbers and tomatoes can increase fluid intake.

Exercise and Activity

Regular physical activity supports not only physical health but also mental well-being, reducing the risk of depression and anxiety. Here are ways to weave activity into daily life:

- Tailored Exercises: Choose activities that match their current physical abilities and interests. This could be as simple as walking in the garden, stretching exercises, or light housekeeping tasks.
- Routine Integration: Incorporate movement into the daily routine. For instance, walking to the mailbox each day or dancing to a favorite song each morning can make exercise a regular, enjoyable part of the day.
- Safety First: Always ensure the environment is safe for physical activity. Remove any tripping hazards and provide sturdy chairs for seated exercises.

Professional Support

There may come a time when the guidance of professionals is beneficial to address specific dietary or physical needs:

- Dietitians: Consulting a dietitian can help tailor eating plans to meet nutritional needs, especially if weight loss or difficulty swallowing becomes a concern.
- Physical Therapists: A physical therapist can create a custom exercise program that considers physical limitations, focusing on maintaining mobility and balance.
- Occupational Therapists: They can offer strategies for making

meal times less stressful and engaging and safe ways to encourage physical activity.

As we tend to the nutritional and physical needs of individuals with dementia, we do more than care for their bodies. We offer them vitality, moments of joy, and an improved quality of life. A balanced diet and regular movement are not just acts of sustenance but of love and care.

By focusing on these areas, we create a nurturing environment that respects their needs and honors their preferences, making every day an opportunity for positive experiences. As we move forward, let's carry with us the understanding that caring for someone with dementia goes beyond meeting basic needs—enriching their lives, one meal and one step at a time.

In conclusion, let's review our care plan and its components. All the details and strategies are already outlined in the chapter. The following table will assist you in making sure everything is on track and that you are not missing any opportunity to improve the care your loved one receives.

CHAPTER 5
CHECKLIST ITEMS

Daily Care Plan Review
Aspect of Care
Checklist Items

M *orning Calmness*

Start the day with a calming activity such as listening to soft music or enjoying a cup of tea together.

Mealtime Regularity

Ensure meals are served at the same time every day to regulate the body's internal clock and contribute to better digestion and overall well-being.

Evening Wind-down

Establish a soothing evening routine such as reading a book or giving a gentle hand massage with lotion to aid in better sleep for both the individual and the caregiver.

Creating a Flexible Schedule

Prioritize important activities and routines for consistency, such as medication times and meals, while allowing flexibility for adaptation to changing needs.

Incorporate periods of rest and unstructured time to accommodate fluctuating energy levels and mood.

Be prepared to modify the day's plan based on the individual's feelings and needs, allowing for both more activities or a slower pace as required.

Involving the Individual

Offer choices within the routine to support autonomy and decision-making skills.

Encourage participation in manageable tasks to boost confidence and provide a sense of purpose.

Pay attention to nonverbal cues to adjust the plan to align more closely with the individual's comfort and enjoyment.

Documentation and Communication

Keep a folder with the daily routine, medication schedule, and pertinent information as a quick reference for all caregivers.

Utilize apps or digital calendars for real-time updates and coordination among family members and caregivers.

Hold regular meetings with family members and other caregivers to discuss the care plan, share observations, and make adjustments as needed.

Make a Difference with Your Review

"The greatest gift you can give to someone is your time, your attention, your love, your concern." - Joel Osteen

Have you seen someone looking lost and confused in a busy city? That could be someone with dementia, a condition that changes lives deeply. We need to understand and help.

Would you help someone you've never met? Our goal with "Understanding Dementia Caregiving Challenges" is to help everyone understand this tough situation better. We need your help to reach more people.

This is where you come in. Reviews are super important. Here's my request for a caregiver you might never meet:

Please take a minute to leave a review for this book.

It doesn't cost you anything but a little bit of time, and it can change someone's life. Your review could empower another family, inspire hope in a caregiver, enhance understanding of dementia, create peaceful homes, and fulfill dreams of better care.

To leave your review, just scan the QR code below:

If you're willing to help someone you've never seen, you're exactly the kind of friend we love. Welcome to our community. You're one of us now.

Thank you from the bottom of my heart. Let's get back to learning more together.

• Your biggest fan, Dean Ramsey

PS - Did you know? When you share something helpful, you become even more special to others. If you think this book could help another caregiver, why not share it with them? Let's spread the kindness and support together.

CHAPTER 7
STEERING THROUGH LEGALITIES

"Kindness can transform someone's dark moment with a blaze of light. You'll never know how much your caring matters." - Amy Leigh Mercree.

Caregiving in dementia is a severe affair; you are responsible for a whole other person, which puts you in a position to protect their rights and authority. Just because they are not in a state to make complex decisions today does not mean that they never were. It is their legal right to be treated with respect and consideration when making decisions for them. This is where legalities come in; honestly, they are not always daunting. They help you in choosing the best for your loved ones. Therefore, legal documents such as wills, advanced directives, and powers of attorney serve distinct purposes in safeguarding the interests and wishes of someone with dementia.

Navigating this legal landscape doesn't just protect them; it provides peace of mind for everyone involved, ensuring that decisions align with their values and desires. So, let's untangle the complexities and set up a system that works seamlessly, ensuring dignity and respect at every turn.

Understanding Legal Documents

Legal documents might seem daunting at first glance. Still, they're essential tools that ensure a person's wishes are honored, especially when they might not be able to articulate them themselves. Here's a breakdown:

- Wills: A will is like a detailed instruction manual for after someone has passed away, specifying how they want their assets distributed and who should be in charge of the process.
- Advanced Directives: These are the pre-set preferences for medical care, often detailing what treatments should or should not be pursued in situations where someone can't make decisions for themselves. It's like setting up your preferences in an app before you start using it.
- Power of Attorney: This grants someone the authority to decide on another's behalf. Think of it as handing over the control of the remote, trusting that they'll make the choices you would have made.

Understanding these documents and ensuring they're in place is like having a safety net and providing clarity and direction during challenging times.

Choosing the Right Power of Attorney

A power of attorney (POA) for a dementia patient is a legal document that grants authority to another person (the agent or attorney-in-fact) to make decisions on behalf of the individual with dementia (the principal) when they are no longer able to make decisions independently due to their cognitive decline. Selecting someone as a power of attorney (POA) involves more than trust; it's about capability and willingness to make hard decisions under pressure. Here are some tips for choosing the right person:

- Consider the Responsibilities: A POA might have to make tough calls, from financial decisions to health-related choices. Ensure the person you're considering understands what's involved and is up to the task.
- Communication Skills: They should be someone who can keep an open line of communication with all parties involved, ensuring transparency and clarity in decision-making.
- Availability: The ideal POA is often someone who can be available to make decisions quickly and efficiently without being hindered by geographical distance or other commitments.

Remember, this choice significantly impacts how effectively your loved one's wishes are honored and how smoothly affairs are managed.

Discussing Wills and Directives

Starting a conversation about wills and advanced directives might feel uncomfortable, but it's critical to ensure everyone's on the same page. Consider these approaches:

- Choose the Right Setting: Pick a calm, quiet time when you won't be rushed or interrupted. This shows respect for the gravity of the conversation.
- Focus on Their Wishes: The goal is to honor their values and desires, making it about safeguarding their wishes rather than focusing on the legalities.
- Involve the Right People: Sometimes, having a neutral third party, like a family lawyer or a trusted friend, can help facilitate the discussion, offering a balanced perspective.

This conversation is about laying the groundwork for future peace of mind, ensuring that decisions made down the line truly reflect your loved one's preferences.

Seeking Legal Advice

Professional guidance is necessary when it comes to setting up legal documents. Here's why:

- Complexity: Laws can vary significantly from one location to another, and the intricacies of legal language can be challenging to navigate without specialized knowledge.
- Updates and Changes: Legal standards and requirements can change. A professional stays abreast of these changes, ensuring documents remain valid and enforceable.
- Personalized Advice: Every situation is unique. A legal professional can offer tailored advice, considering all aspects of your loved one's circumstances and wishes.

Finding a lawyer specializing in elder law can make this process smoother, offering expertise that aligns with the specific needs and challenges of dementia care.

In summary, steering through the legal aspects of dementia care involves understanding the purpose and importance of critical documents, choosing the right people to entrust decision-making roles, and seeking professional advice to navigate the complexities involved.

Financial Strategies: Managing the Costs of Dementia Care

When facing the financial realities of dementia care, envisioning a future where your loved one's needs are fully met without compromising financial stability can feel like navigating through a dense fog. However, with the right strategies, the path can become apparent. Crafting a budget, exploring insurance options, planning for the long term, and steering clear of financial pitfalls are like setting up beacons.

Budgeting for Dementia Care

The budget includes predictable expenses like ongoing medical care and less predictable ones like home modifications or emergency care needs. How well you plan and manage your budget directly decides the quality of care you can provide. Therefore, it should consider all aspects of dementia care discussed in previous chapters. Here's how to start:

- List All Potential Costs: Gather information on all possible expenses, from daily care needs to potential future costs. Don't forget about the less obvious ones, like transportation for medical appointments.
- Track Spending: Use apps or a simple spreadsheet to monitor expenses over a few months. This snapshot of where money is going helps identify areas for adjustments.
- Allocate Funds: Based on your tracking, allocate funds to different categories. Prioritize essential expenses and see where there might be room to save.

Exploring Insurance Options

Diving into the insurance world to find coverage that aligns with the needs of someone with dementia is crucial. It's not just about having insurance but having the right insurance. Consider these steps:

- Review Current Policies: Look closely at existing health or disability insurance policies to understand what aspects of dementia care are covered.
- Long-term Care Insurance: If not already in place, explore long-term care insurance options. These policies can significantly offset the costs of home care services, assisted living, and other long-term care facilities.
- Life Insurance Policies: Some life insurance policies offer an accelerated death benefit, providing a cash advance on the death benefit to cover costs related to long-term care.

Planning for the Long Term

Setting up a long-term financial plan is much like planting a tree. It's an investment in the future, ensuring that resources will be available when needed. Here's how to nurture this financial growth:

- Savings and Investments: If possible, save for future care needs. Consider talking to a financial advisor about investment options that offer growth or income.
- Special Needs Trust: This is a legal arrangement where funds are set aside to benefit someone with a disability without affecting their eligibility for public assistance programs. It ensures that resources are managed and used according to the family's wishes, providing for the loved one's needs in the coming years.
- Government Benefits: Look into eligibility for government programs that can help support long-term care costs. While navigating these waters can be complex, the potential financial support is worth the effort.

Avoiding Common Financial Pitfalls

Navigating financial management for a loved one with dementia also means being vigilant about potential pitfalls and scams that target the elderly. Here are ways to safeguard against these threats:

- Stay Informed: Educate yourself about common scams and financial risks facing seniors. Knowledge is power when it comes to prevention.
- Secure Personal Information: Ensure that sensitive financial information, online accounts, and personal documents are secured. Consider a lockbox or a digital password manager.
- Regular Financial Reviews: Make it a habit to review bank statements, credit card statements, and other financial documents regularly for any unusual activity.

- Professional Advice: When in doubt, seek advice from financial advisors or legal professionals specializing in elder law. They can offer strategies for protecting assets and ensuring economic security.

If you find yourself overwhelmed by the finances, seek the help of another family member in financial management. Once again, knowledge is power. The more you know about the healthcare, legal, and financial systems, the better you can plan and manage your budget. So, telling another soul in your support network may open a door for you to overcome your barriers. Usually, dementia support networks also share tips and guidelines about the financial aspects of dementia care, so attending educational events would be a great help.

Government Aid and Insurance

In dementia care, understanding and accessing government aid and insurance is foundational. These resources can offer a lifeline, providing financial backing and services essential for comprehensive care. However, like all governmental procedures, this can also be confusing. So, let's simplify it.

Medicare and Medicaid

At the heart of government assistance for seniors are Medicare and Medicaid, two programs that, while distinct, offer critical support for individuals with dementia.

- Medicare primarily serves individuals over 65, offering coverage that includes hospital stays, medical visits, and, in some instances, short-term home health services or rehabilitation. However, it's vital to note that Medicare's coverage of long-term care services is limited. For dementia care, Medicare may cover diagnostic evaluations, some medications, and occupational therapies. Applying for

Medicare is straightforward and can be done online at the Social Security Administration's website or in person at a local office.

- Medicaid, on the other hand, extends its hand to those with limited income and resources. Unlike Medicare, Medicaid can cover long-term care, including nursing home services and, in some states, home and community-based services. Each state operates its Medicaid program within federal guidelines so that coverage can vary. To apply for Medicaid, contact your state's Medicaid office. Preparation is vital; gather financial documents and medical records before initiating the application process.

Veterans Benefits

For those who served, veterans' benefits shine as beacons of hope, offering additional support that can significantly ease the financial burden of dementia care.

- For example, the Aid and Attendance benefit provides monthly payments on top of the regular pension for veterans and surviving spouses who require assistance with daily activities. Qualifying for this benefit involves meeting specific service and financial criteria.
- The Veterans Directed Care program offers another support layer, allowing veterans to manage their care services directly, tailoring them to their specific needs. This program emphasizes autonomy and personalization in care.

Accessing these benefits starts with a visit to the Veterans Affairs (VA) website or a local VA office. The process can be complicated, requiring detailed service records and medical documentation, but the potential relief it brings is substantial.

State and Local Programs

Dotted across the landscape of dementia care are state and local programs designed to support individuals and their caregivers. These can range from respite care services, offering caregivers a much-needed break, to adult day care programs that provide social and health services.

- A good starting point for tapping into these resources is your local Area Agency on Aging (AAA). AAAs are invaluable in pointing families toward programs and services tailored to their needs.
- Additionally, many states offer waiver programs that provide financial assistance for home and community-based services, helping individuals with dementia remain in their homes for as long as possible.

Finding these programs often requires some detective work, but the effort can uncover valuable resources that lighten the load of dementia care.

Utilizing Social Workers

Social workers emerge as guides in navigating government aid and insurance, illuminating paths families might not have found on their own. These are the right people with the proper knowledge and intentions. They make everything a whole lot easier. Here's what you need to know:

- Social workers specialize in connecting individuals with resources, understanding the intricacies of application processes, and advocating for the needs of those in their care.
- They can assist in evaluating eligibility for various programs, filling out necessary paperwork, and even addressing potential roadblocks along the way.

- Many hospitals, clinics, and community centers have social workers on staff. Don't hesitate to ask for their assistance or for recommendations on where to find one in your community.

These steps not only help mitigate the financial challenges associated with dementia care but also ensure that individuals have access to the comprehensive services they need to navigate their daily lives with dignity and comfort.

Long-Term Care Options: Making Informed Choices

Choosing the proper care setting for a loved one with dementia is a decision that weighs heavily on many families. It's about balancing the need for specialized care and the desire to maintain as much normalcy and comfort as possible. From the cozy familiarity of at-home care to the comprehensive support offered in assisted living and nursing homes, each option carries its own considerations.

Types of Long-Term Care

- At-home care allows individuals to stay in a familiar environment, surrounded by possessions and memories. Home health aides can provide personalized care, from assistance with daily activities to medical support.
- Assisted Living Facilities offer a blend of independence and care. Residents live in apartments but can access assistance, meals, and social activities. These facilities often have specialized units for dementia care.
- Nursing Homes provide the most comprehensive level of care, including 24-hour medical supervision and assistance with all aspects of daily life. They're suitable for individuals with advanced dementia who need extensive support.

Evaluating these options means weighing the benefits of each against the specific needs and preferences of your loved one. Once again, it helps to note all the details in a journal and consult a professional.

Evaluating Care Facilities

Finding a suitable facility involves more than ticking boxes for services and amenities. Consider these factors:

- Staff-to-Resident Ratio: High staffing levels mean more personalized attention and care.
- Dementia Care Expertise: Facilities with specialized dementia care units or staff trained in dementia care can offer a more supportive environment for your loved one.
- Activities and Engagement: Look for programs that engage residents in meaningful activities tailored to their abilities and interests.
- Feedback from Current Residents and Families: Conversations with current residents or their families can provide insight into the facility's quality of care and life.

Ideally, visiting potential facilities multiple times during different parts of the day can help you get a feel for the environment and how residents are treated.

The Transition to Long-Term Care

Moving a loved one into long-term care is a significant change that can stir up a mix of emotions for everyone involved. Here's how to ease the transition:

- Involve Your Loved One: As much as possible, involve them in discussions about their care. Even if making the final choice isn't feasible, small decisions about their new space can make them feel part of the process.
- Personalize Their Space: Bring items from home to make their new environment feel familiar and comforting.
- Frequent Visits: Regular visits can ease the sense of separation and help your loved one adjust to their new surroundings.

Adjusting to this period is natural, and patience is key as everyone adapts to the new living arrangement. Describing it as "painful" is an understatement, so holding onto your inner strength during these times is crucial. Ensure that you've made the right decisions and that this is precisely what your loved one needs. Knowing that you prioritize the best care for them can help reconcile thoughts and emotions.

Maintaining Connection

Preserving the bond with your loved one after they move into long-term care is crucial for their well-being and yours. Here are ways to stay involved:

- Establish a Visiting Routine: Regular visits can provide comfort and continuity. Engaging in activities together during visits can also enhance your connection.
- Participate in Care Planning: Stay involved in your loved one's care decisions. Attending care plan meetings allows you to advocate for their needs and preferences.
- Use Technology: Video calls and digital photo frames can help you stay connected between visits, sharing moments and memories even when apart.

Maintaining a solid connection ensures that your loved one continues to feel valued and loved, reinforcing the importance of family and familiar relationships in their care.

As we wrap up this exploration of long-term care options for individuals with dementia, it's clear that each family's path will be unique, guided by the specific needs, preferences, and circumstances of their loved one. From the intimate setting of at-home care to the comprehensive support of nursing homes, the goal remains: to provide a safe, nurturing environment where our loved ones can live with dignity. Making informed choices about long-term care, preparing for the transition, and maintaining a close connection affirm our commitment to their well-being. As we move forward, let's carry with us the understanding that even as care needs evolve, our relationship's essence and dedication to those we care for remain unwavering.

CHAPTER 8

EMOTIONAL RESILIENCE

"The oak fought the wind and was broken, the willow bent when it must and survived." - Robert Jordan.

C aring for someone with dementia is like trying to piece together a puzzle without the picture on the box. It's challenging, sometimes confusing, but also deeply rewarding. Emotions run high within this maze of responsibilities, and stress can become a constant companion. A child may feel guilty for not being able to support their parent by themselves and having to rely on other caregivers; a partner may feel lonely and grieve their companionship; a sibling may feel weary and heartbroken. There are as many scenarios as there are people with dementia with their loved ones taking care of them. You, my readers, are among these people, and you must face your unique internal challenges. It is often easier to bear financial troubles and make up for any resource constraints, but it is an entirely different battle on the inside. Managing the deluge of emotions is the most courageous bit, which is often invisible to the naked eye.

In this chapter, I will make a humble effort to share the tools and techniques to manage stress, fostering emotional resilience that sustains both you and your loved one through this experience.

Identifying and Managing Stress

Stress doesn't always announce itself with a loud bang. Often, the quiet accumulation of daily frustrations, constant worry, or the physical demands of caregiving weigh us down. Recognizing these sources is the first step toward managing them. Consider keeping a stress diary for a week. Note moments when you feel overwhelmed, what triggered these feelings, and how you responded. You might find patterns that point to specific stressors, be it lack of sleep, financial worries, or the emotional toll of seeing your loved one's condition change.

Developing Coping Mechanisms

Once you've pinpointed the sources of your stress, you can start building your toolkit of coping mechanisms. Here are some strategies that have proven effective:

- Mindfulness and Meditation: These practices help center your thoughts and reduce anxiety. Even five minutes a day can make a difference. There are plenty of free apps and online resources to get you started.
- Respite Care: Taking a break is not a luxury—it's a necessity. Look into local respite care services where your loved one can be safely cared for while you recharge. Sometimes, a few hours a week can provide the breather you need.
- Physical Activity: Exercise releases endorphins, the body's natural stress-relievers. You don't need to commit to a rigorous workout routine; a daily walk, gardening, or gentle yoga can boost your mood and energy levels.
- Hobbies and Social Interactions: Reconnecting with activities you love and spending time with friends can remind you of

life outside caregiving. It's essential to maintain these connections for your emotional well-being.

Seeking Professional Help

There's strength in recognizing when you need support beyond what friends, family, or self-care can provide. If stress feels unmanageable, consider seeking help from a professional. This could mean talking to a counselor specializing in caregiver stress or joining a support group where you can share experiences and strategies with others in similar situations. Remember, asking for help reflects your commitment to providing the best care possible, not just for your loved one but for yourself as well.

Forming a Self-Care Routine

Self-care isn't a one-time activity; it's a routine that maintains your well-being. Here are some ideas to build your self-care routine:

- Schedule It: Just as you schedule appointments for your loved one, make self-care a non-negotiable part of your calendar. Please treat it with the same importance, whether it's a hobby, exercise, or quiet time.
- Sleep and Nutrition: Prioritize good sleep hygiene and nourishing foods. These basic steps can significantly impact your ability to cope with stress.
- Stay Connected: Keep in touch with friends and family. Social connections can provide emotional support and moments of joy amid challenging times.
- Reflect and Adjust: Regularly review your self-care routine. What's working? What isn't? Adjust as needed to find what best supports your resilience.
- Mindfulness in Action: Try eating one meal a day mindfully. Turn off the TV, put away the phone, and focus solely on the experience of eating. Notice the colors, textures, and flavors. This practice can be a simple, daily reminder to stay present.

- Exercise Buddy: Partner with a friend or another caregiver for regular walks. This combines physical activity with social interaction, doubling the stress-relieving benefits.
- Journaling: End each day with a gratitude journal. Writing down even small things you're thankful for can shift focus from the day's challenges to blessings.
- Stress Diary Template: Start with a simple notebook or use a digital app to track your reactions to stressors.
- Meditation Guides: Look for beginner-friendly meditation guides or apps that offer short, daily practices.
- Physical Activity Log: Keep track of your daily activities. Set realistic goals and celebrate when you meet them.
- Respite Care Directory: Compile a list of local respite care services. Include contact information, services offered, and any costs involved.

Building resilience isn't about avoiding stress but handling it gracefully. By identifying stressors, employing coping strategies, seeking help when needed, and establishing a self-care routine, you're not just surviving the caregiving experience but thriving within it.

Grieving in Advance: Navigating Anticipatory Grief and Loss

Anticipatory grief is a unique and profound sorrow experienced before an impending loss, particularly prevalent in caregivers of individuals with dementia. This form of grief can be as intense and overwhelming as the grief felt after a loss, sometimes even more so, because it involves grieving someone who is still alive. It's a complex mix of emotions, including sadness, loss, guilt, and sometimes relief, all of which can occur in anticipation of the final goodbye.

Understanding Anticipatory Grief

Anticipatory grief might manifest in various ways, such as sadness at the thought of future loss, anxiety about what the final stages of dementia might bring, or guilt over feeling relief at moments when caregiving becomes especially burdensome. For many, it's mourning the progressive loss of the person they once knew, even as they continue to care for them. Recognizing this grief is crucial, as it validates the caregiver's feelings and helps them understand that what they're experiencing is a normal, albeit heart-wrenching, part of the caregiving process.

Coping Strategies

Dealing with anticipatory grief demands a gentle approach, one that acknowledges the pain while finding ways to manage it:

- Seek Support: Connecting with others who understand what you're going through can be incredibly comforting. Support groups, either in-person or online, can offer a space to share your feelings and learn from others on a similar path.
- Express Emotions: Keeping a journal, creating art, or engaging in other forms of self-expression can provide an outlet for your grief. Writing letters to your loved one, even if they're never sent, can also be a therapeutic way to articulate your feelings.
- Cherish Quality Time: Focus on creating moments of connection with your loved one, no matter how small. Simple activities like looking through photo albums, listening to their favorite music, or enjoying nature together can bring joy and comfort to both of you.
- Self-Care: Remember to take care of yourself. Eating well, getting enough rest, and finding time for activities you enjoy are vital for maintaining your strength during this challenging time.

Preparing for the Future

Facing what lies ahead can help you feel more prepared when the time comes. Some steps include:

- Understanding the Disease's Progression: Educating yourself about the stages of dementia can help you anticipate changes in your loved one's condition and care needs.
- Making Legal and Financial Arrangements: Ensuring that wills, advanced directives, and financial plans are in order can relieve some of the stress and uncertainty about the future.
- Discussing Wishes and Preferences: Conversations with your loved one about their wishes for end-of-life care, while challenging, can ensure that their preferences are honored and provide you with a sense of peace.

Finding Meaning

Amid grief, finding meaning in the caregiving experience can offer solace and a sense of purpose. Consider:

- Reflecting on the Journey: Take time to reflect on the journey you and your loved one have shared. Acknowledge the love, the challenges, and the growth you've experienced along the way.
- Honoring Their Legacy: Think about ways to honor your loved one's life and legacy, such as compiling a memory book or organizing a charitable event in their name.
- Seeking Personal Growth: Many caregivers find that their experience leads to personal growth, whether developing greater empathy, strength, or an appreciation for the fragility of life.

Feeling anticipatory grief and loss is an intensely personal process, one that unfolds differently for everyone. It involves not only mourning the impending loss of a loved one but also coming to terms with the gradual changes dementia brings. Caregivers can forge a path through these difficult emotions by understanding anticipatory grief, employing coping strategies, preparing for the future, and finding meaning in the experience. This approach allows for moments of beauty and connection amidst the sorrow, offering a reminder that love endures even in the face of loss.

Finding Joy in the Journey

How could someone find joy in loss? It seems paradoxical. Yet, caregiving for dementia brings such poignant moments that allow for meaningful experiences. It may not be the fun we are used to, but it brings tremendous and deep-felt joy when we share moments with our loved ones. These are our windows to heaven, which soothe the mind and heart and make it clear that our caregiving has purpose and meaning and that we are indeed making a difference.

Celebrating Small Victories

In dementia care, small victories hold profound significance. A shared laugh, a moment of recognition, or a successful completion of a simple task—these are milestones worth celebrating. They remind us of the resilience and enduring spirit of our loved ones, offering glimpses of their essence that dementia cannot dim. Acknowledging these victories uplifts the spirits of both caregiver and recipient, reinforcing the value of our efforts and the impact of our care.

- Record these moments, perhaps in a journal or a digital album, creating a collection of joyful memories.
- Share these victories with friends and family, spreading the joy and fostering a broader appreciation for the positive moments.

Creating New Memories

The progression of dementia might alter how we create memories, but it doesn't halt the process. Every interaction holds the potential for new, meaningful experiences that enrich our connection with our loved ones.

- Engage in activities that resonate with your loved one's interests and abilities. Simple crafts, listening to music, or enjoying nature can be sources of joy and new memories.
- Capture these moments through photos or short videos, creating tangible reminders of the joy shared.

Maintaining a Sense of Humor

"Humor is the great thing, the saving thing after all. The minute it crops up, all our hardnesses yield, all our irritations and resentments flit away, and a sunny spirit takes their place." – *Mark Twain.*

Humor is a powerful tool in dealing with challenges. It provides relief, fosters connection, and brings lightness to situations that might otherwise feel heavy. A shared laugh can bridge the gap dementia creates, reminding us of the joy in our relationships.

- Find humor in the daily mishaps and unexpected moments. Laughter can be a shared language, transcending the barriers dementia might impose.
- Watch comedies or share funny stories. These moments of shared amusement can deeply bond, offering respite from the daily challenges.

Ultimately, the essence of our caregiving journey lies in enhancing the quality of life for our loved ones and ourselves. Living in the moment becomes not just a strategy but a way of life, where each day is an opportunity to find joy, connection, and fulfillment. Prioritize activities that bring pleasure and relaxation to your loved one, tailoring your approach to their evolving preferences and abilities. Create an environment that stimulates the senses and fosters comfort, using music, art, and nature to enrich the daily experience. Embrace flexibility, allowing for spontaneous moments of joy and connection that arise from simply being together.

As we close this chapter, we carry with us the understanding that amidst the intricacies of dementia care, there are endless opportunities for joy, laughter, and meaningful experiences. By celebrating small victories, creating new memories, maintaining a sense of humor, and focusing on the quality of life, we honor the journey of our loved ones and ourselves. These principles guide us through the present and pave the way for continued growth and fulfillment as we move forward into the next phase of our caregiving journey.

CHAPTER 9

WHEN HOME CARE ISN'T ENOUGH

In the end, it's not the years in your life that count. It's the life in your years. — Abraham Lincoln.

I magine sitting at a familiar dinner table, but tonight, the chair across from you is empty. It's a jarring sight that starkly reminds you of the shifts happening right before your eyes. This moment, though simple, can be an unsettling wake-up call, signaling that the care needs of your loved one with dementia might have outgrown the bounds of home.

Deciding to transition from home care to professional care is no small task. It's filled with emotional weight and practical considerations, each demanding attention and care. This chapter aims to shed light on the signs that indicate a move might be necessary and how to approach this transition with knowledge and empathy.

Assessing Care Needs

Recognizing when home care is insufficient hinges on a clear-eyed assessment of your loved one's needs. It's like looking at the fuel gauge on a long road trip; you need to know how much gas you have to decide if it's time to refuel. Here are steps to help gauge the situation:

- Daily Living Activities: Take note of changes in their ability to perform daily tasks, such as dressing, bathing, and eating. It might be time to consider additional support when these become overwhelmingly challenging.
- Safety Concerns: Assess the home for potential safety hazards. Frequent falls, difficulty navigating stairs, or forgetting to turn off appliances can all signal that a safer environment is needed.
- Caregiver Capacity: Reflect honestly on your ability to provide care. If you find yourself stretched thin, battling chronic fatigue, or feeling emotionally drained, it may be beneficial for both you and your loved one to explore professional care options.

Behavioral and Medical Indicators

Sometimes, specific behavioral or medical changes signal the need for a transition to professional care. These indicators can serve as clear signs that more specialized care is needed:

- Escalating Behavioral Issues: If your loved one exhibits increased aggression, wandering, or severe anxiety, it might be beyond what home care can effectively manage.
- Complex Medical Needs: The emergence of medical conditions that require regular monitoring by healthcare professionals or specialized equipment not feasible at home can necessitate a move to a facility with 24/7 care.

Family Dynamics and Caregiver Burnout

The ripple effects of dementia care extend beyond the individual to touch the whole family. It's important to consider how the caregiving situation affects family dynamics and the health of the caregiver:

- Family Stress: Pay attention to signs of stress or strain among other family members. Persistent tension, arguments over care decisions, or withdrawal from family activities can all be indicators that the current care situation is unsustainable.
- Caregiver Health: If you, as the primary caregiver, find your health deteriorating—lost sleep, skipped meals, or ignored medical appointments—it's a stark indicator that the current arrangement might not be tenable in the long term.

Consulting with Healthcare Professionals

In navigating these waters, healthcare professionals can offer invaluable guidance. They bring an outside perspective, grounded in medical expertise, to help assess your loved one's needs:

- Regular Check-ups: Use regular medical check-ups to discuss your observations and concerns about your loved one's condition and care needs.
- Seek Specialized Advice: Consider consulting professionals who specialize in dementia care. They can provide insights into your loved one's condition and offer recommendations on the type of care facility that would best meet their needs.
- Care Manager Consultation: A care manager, often a nurse or social worker, can assess your loved one's situation, suggest care options, and help navigate the transition to professional care. They can be a bridge between you, your loved one, and potential care facilities.

As you find yourself at this crossroads, remember that shifting to professional care doesn't diminish the love or commitment you've shown. It's simply acknowledging that the care landscape has changed, and it's time to adjust the sails to ensure your loved one continues to receive the best care possible. This decision, though difficult, is made from a place of deep love and respect for their well-being and dignity.

Choosing the Right Facility: What to Look For

Selecting a care facility for a loved one affected by dementia is akin to finding a new home that's not just safe and comfortable but also nurturing and engaging. It's a decision that involves more than just ticking boxes for amenities; it's about finding a place where your loved one will feel respected, understood, and cared for.

Before you move forward, I suggest opening that journal where you jot down important things and make your notes as you read. Let's explore the steps to make this crucial decision a bit easier.

Types of Care Facilities

Facilities offering care for individuals with dementia vary widely, each tailored to meet different levels of care needs:

- Assisted Living Facilities provide a residential setting with personal care support, meals, and health services. These are ideal for relatively independent individuals who require assistance with daily tasks.
- Skilled Nursing Facilities offer a higher level of medical care. Staffed with healthcare professionals, they cater to residents needing 24-hour monitoring and medical care.
- Memory Care Units specialize in caring for those with Alzheimer's and other dementias. With secure environments and staff trained in dementia care, they focus on enhancing the quality of life for residents with cognitive impairments.
- Continuing Care Retirement Communities offer a spectrum of care from independent living to skilled nursing care, allowing residents to transition between levels of care as needed.

Each type of facility offers unique benefits, and the choice largely depends on the specific care needs and preferences of your loved one.

Important Facility Criteria

When evaluating facilities, certain criteria stand out as particularly crucial for ensuring the well-being of your loved one:

- Staff Qualifications and Training: Ensure the staff is qualified and has specific training in dementia care, understanding the unique needs and behaviors associated with the condition.
- Resident-to-Staff Ratio: A lower ratio means more personalized care and attention, which is vital for individuals with dementia who may require more time and patience from caregivers.
- Dementia-Specific Care Programs: Look for facilities that offer programs and activities designed to engage residents with dementia, promoting cognitive function and social interaction.
- Safety and Security: Facilities should have measures in place to ensure the safety of residents, especially those prone to wandering, including secure outdoor spaces and monitoring systems.

Visiting and Evaluating Facilities

Visiting potential facilities gives you insight into the daily life and atmosphere of the place. Here are some tips for making the most of your visits:

- Schedule Multiple Visits: Visit at different times of the day to get a sense of the daily routine, how the staff interacts with residents, and the overall atmosphere.
- Prepare Questions: Ask about staff training, the ratio of staff to residents, how they handle medical emergencies, and what a typical day looks like for a resident.
- Observe Interactions: Pay attention to how staff interacts with

residents. Are they patient and respectful? Do residents seem engaged and content?

- Check for Cleanliness: The facility should be clean and well-maintained, with no unpleasant odors or unattended hazards.
- Meal Quality: If possible, arrange a meal during your visit. The quality and variety of food and the dining experience are important aspects of daily life in the facility.

Involving Your Loved One

While dementia might limit your loved one's ability to participate fully in the decision-making process, involving them as much as possible respects their dignity and preferences:

- Discuss Options: Share information about the facilities you're considering. If they can, involve them in discussions about what they would prefer regarding living arrangements.
- Visit Together: If feasible, bring your loved one to visit potential facilities. Please pay attention to their reactions and comfort level.
- Consider Their Preferences: Reflect on what you know about their preferences and personality. Would they thrive in a larger community with many activities or prefer a quieter, more intimate setting?

In the end, choosing a suitable facility is a profoundly personal decision, influenced by the unique needs and personality of your loved one. By carefully considering the types of facilities available, evaluating them based on critical criteria, involving your loved one in the process, and trusting your instincts, you can find a place where they will be cared for and cherished.

Making the Transition: Tips for a Smooth Move

Moving a loved one with dementia into a care facility is a significant step, marked by a mix of emotions and practical challenges. Let me share some guidance on ensuring a gentle transition, focusing on preparation, personalizing the new space, navigating the initial weeks, and supporting your loved one through this change.

Preparation is Key

Starting conversations early and framing them in positive, reassuring language can help ease the path for your loved one. Here's how you might approach this:

- Early Conversations: Discuss the idea of moving well before the day arrives. Use simple, straightforward language to explain the reasons, focusing on the positives.
- Involvement in Choices: If possible, involve your loved one in decisions about the move. This could be as simple as choosing which items to take with them or selecting room colors.
- Familiarization Visits: Arrange visits to the new facility before the move. This can help your loved one become accustomed to the new surroundings and the people they will be interacting with regularly.

Personalizing the New Space

Creating a familiar and comforting environment in their new living space can significantly impact your loved one's sense of security and well-being.

- Bring Personal Items: Decorate their room with personal items from home—photos, a favorite blanket, or a well-loved piece of furniture. These touches can make the new space feel more like home.
- Create a Memory Box: Fill a box with keepsakes and items that hold special memories for your loved one. This can serve as a comforting link to their past.
- Sensory Comforts: Incorporate items that engage the senses,

such as a scented diffuser with a familiar fragrance or a playlist of their favorite music.

The First Few Weeks

The initial period after the move is crucial for helping your loved one adjust to their new environment. Here are some strategies to navigate this time:

- Frequent Visits: Initially, visit often to provide a sense of continuity and reassurance. However, be mindful of your loved one's cues; too much change at once can be overwhelming.
- Establish a Routine: Work with the care facility staff to establish a daily routine similar to what your loved one was accustomed to at home. Familiar routines can provide comfort and stability.
- Open Communication with Staff: Maintain open lines of communication with the facility's staff. Share insights about your loved one's likes, dislikes, and what comforts them. This information can help staff provide more personalized care.

Supporting Emotional Adjustment

Adjusting to a new living situation takes time, and it's natural for your loved one to experience a range of emotions. Here are ways you can support them through this adjustment period:

- Validate Feelings: Acknowledge your loved one's feelings about the move. They must know feeling uncertain or sad about the changes is okay.
- Encourage Socialization: Gently encourage your loved one to participate in activities and social events at the facility. Making new friends and finding enjoyable activities can ease the transition.

- Monitor Well-being: Keep a close eye on your loved one's emotional and physical well-being during the initial weeks. Regularly check in with them and the care staff to ensure their needs are being met.

Moving a loved one with dementia into a care facility is a profound change for everyone involved. With thoughtful preparation, personal touches to make the new space feel like home, careful navigation of the first few weeks, and supportive strategies for emotional adjustment, you can help make this transition as smooth and comforting as possible. Through this process, remember that your support and love remain constant, providing a reassuring presence as your loved one adapts to their new environment.

Staying Involved and Aware of the Care Facility

Moving a loved one into a care facility doesn't mean stepping back from their life—it means changing how you're involved. And there are undoubtedly many more fronts where you are needed once your loved one enters a care facility. You even get the chance to stay aware of the care facility practices for the sake of your loved one and for every other patient who resides there; your duties almost transition from personal to social.

Building Relationships with Staff

A positive rapport with the staff at a care facility can significantly enhance the quality of care your loved one receives. Here are some strategies to foster these essential connections:

- Initial Introductions: Make an effort to meet the staff members directly involved in your loved one's care. Understanding their roles and expressing appreciation for their work can lay a strong foundation for a collaborative relationship.
- Regular, Open Communication: Establish a routine for regular updates on your loved one's condition and care. Whether

through scheduled meetings, email updates, or informal chats, consistent communication helps you stay informed and involved.

- Express Concerns Respectfully: If you have concerns, address them directly but respectfully with the staff. Framing concerns as questions rather than accusations can lead to more productive conversations and solutions.

Monitoring Care Quality

Staying vigilant about the care your loved one receives is crucial. Here's how you can effectively monitor their care:

- Personal Observations: During visits, pay close attention to your loved one's physical appearance, mood, and the cleanliness of their environment. Changes in these areas can be early indicators of issues.
- Feedback from Your Loved One: If they can, ask your loved one about their experiences and feelings regarding the care they're receiving. Their insights can provide valuable perspectives.
- Review Care Plans: Regularly review your loved one's care plan to ensure it's being followed and updated as their needs change. Don't hesitate to ask for modifications if necessary.

If concerns about care quality arise, here's a pathway to address them:

1. Speak to Staff: If appropriate, address issues with the caregiver or staff member involved.
2. Escalate to Management: If the issue isn't resolved, bring it to the attention of the facility's management.
3. Outside Assistance: Consider seeking assistance from a patient advocate or ombudsman specializing in elder care for unresolved issues.

Effective Advocacy

Advocating for your loved one means being their voice and protector within the care system. Here are some tips to be an effective advocate:

- Educate Yourself: The more you know about dementia and your loved one's rights within a care facility, the better equipped you'll be to advocate for their needs.
- Document Everything: Keep detailed records of conversations, care plans, and incidents. This documentation can be invaluable if issues need to be escalated.
- Build Alliances: Forming positive relationships with staff doesn't just improve daily care; it also means you have allies within the facility who can support your advocacy efforts.

Legal Considerations

We have discussed the legalities of caregiving before, yet some important aspects arise once a care facility becomes part of the process. Understanding and managing legal tools can ensure your loved one's wishes are honored and their rights protected:

- Power of Attorney (POA): If you're designated as a POA, you have the legal authority to make decisions on behalf of your loved one. This role might cover financial matters, healthcare decisions, or both, depending on how the POA is structured. Ensure the care facility has a current copy of this document and understands its implications.
- Guardianship: In situations where a loved one hasn't designated a POA and is unable to make informed decisions, seeking guardianship might be necessary. This legal process grants you the authority to make decisions on their behalf. Consulting with an attorney specializing in elder law can guide you through this complex process.
- Resident Rights: Familiarize yourself with the rights of residents in care facilities. These rights cover a range of

aspects, from the right to privacy and dignity to the right to be informed about care plans and treatments. Understanding these rights can empower you to ensure they're being respected.

In professional care, your involvement and advocacy are pivotal in ensuring your loved one receives the care and respect they deserve. From building relationships with the staff and monitoring the quality of care to navigating legal considerations and advocating effectively, your actions can make a significant difference in your loved one's life. It's about shifting your role from a day-to-day caregiver to an informed, involved advocate who ensures their well-being in a professional care setting.

Adjusting to New Care Dynamics

Moving a loved one into professional care significantly shifts the caregiving landscape. It's a time filled with mixed emotions, from relief to sorrow, and a period that demands adaptation. Here, we'll explore how to navigate these changes, offering strategies to manage the complex feelings that come with them, redefine the caregiver role, seek out support networks, and fully embrace this new chapter of care.

Managing Guilt and Grief

It's natural to grapple with feelings of guilt or grief as your loved one transitions to professional care. You might wonder if you've done enough or mourn the loss of your day-to-day involvement in their care. Here are a few strategies to help process these emotions:

- Acknowledge Your Feelings: Allow yourself to feel whatever emotions arise. Understanding that these feelings are a normal part of the process can be comforting.
- Speak About Your Feelings: Sharing your thoughts with trusted friends, family, or professionals can provide a different perspective and alleviate the burden of guilt.

- Reframe Your Thoughts: Remind yourself that choosing professional care was a decision made out of love and the desire to provide the best possible care for your loved one.

Adjusting to the Caregiver Role

As your loved one settles into a care facility, your role as a caregiver transforms. No longer the primary provider of day-to-day care, you might find yourself searching for how to remain involved. Here's how you might navigate this shift:

- Focus on Advocacy: Your role now includes advocating for your loved one, ensuring their needs and preferences are respected in the care facility.
- Maintain Regular Visits: Maintaining a consistent presence in your loved one's life is vital. These visits can help sustain your bond and comfort both of you.
- Participate in Care Planning: Stay engaged in discussions about your loved one's care plan. Your insights are invaluable in tailoring their care to their unique needs and history.

Finding Support

This transition period is also a time to bolster your support system. Leaning on others can provide emotional relief and practical advice. Here's how to find the support you need:

- Join Support Groups: Connecting with others in similar situations can offer comfort and practical advice. These groups provide a space to share experiences and coping strategies.
- Consider Professional Help: If you find the transition particularly challenging, speaking with a counselor or therapist can provide professional guidance and support.
- Reach Out to Friends and Family: Don't underestimate the power of your existing network. Friends and family can offer a listening ear and help you navigate this change.

Embracing the New Normal

While this transition period can be challenging, it also opens up new possibilities for you and your loved one. Embracing this change involves focusing on the positive aspects:

- Recognize the Benefits: Professional care facilities offer specialized care and social opportunities to significantly enhance your loved one's quality of life.
- Rediscover Personal Time: With reduced day-to-day caregiving responsibilities, you can engage in self-care and revisit personal interests or hobbies.
- Celebrate the Continued Bond: Your relationship with your loved one can continue to grow and evolve, even within the context of professional care. Finding new ways to connect and share can be deeply rewarding.

In closing, let's carry with us the understanding that each step in this journey, no matter how challenging, is taken out of love. It's a testament to our commitment to ensuring the best possible care for our loved ones as we move towards a future that, while different, is still filled with moments of connection, joy, and love.

As we turn the page, we'll explore further how to enhance the lives of those with dementia, ensuring they continue to experience joy, dignity, and a sense of belonging in every stage of their journey.

CHAPTER 10

EMBRACING THE TWILIGHT

"You matter because you are you, and you matter to the end of your life. We will do all we can not only to help you die peacefully but also to live until you die." - Dame Cicely Saunders.

With its warm golden hues, the late afternoon sun softly blankets everything it touches, bringing a serene glow to the end of the day. This time, often referred to as the "golden hour" in photography, is cherished for its ability to cast the world in a gentle, forgiving light. The final stages of dementia can also be seen through a lens of profound, albeit bittersweet, beauty like that of a golden hour. It's a phase where moments of connection, despite their rarity, shine brightly against the backdrop of challenges. In this chapter, we'll navigate the delicate balance of honoring our loved ones' wishes while ensuring comfort and dignity during their twilight days.

Understanding the Final Stages

As dementia progresses, medical and behavioral changes become more pronounced. Recognizing these signs prepares us for the road ahead and guides us in making decisions that align with our loved ones' values and desires. Some common changes include increased difficulty in communicating, a greater need for assistance with daily activities, and shifts in personality and behavior that may require specialized care approaches.

Care Options

When considering care in the final stages, the spectrum of options varies widely, each with its own set of benefits designed to meet the evolving needs of those with advanced dementia. Here's a breakdown:

- Continued Care in a Facility: For many, the transition has already been made to a setting where 24/7 care is available. Ensuring that this environment continues to meet their needs involves regular assessments and open dialogue with care providers.
- Hospice Care: This option focuses on comfort and quality of life rather than curative treatment. Available both in-home and in certain facilities, hospice care supports not just the individual with dementia but also their family, offering medical, emotional, and spiritual resources.
- At-Home Care with Increased Support: Some families choose to keep their loved ones at home, increasing in-home support services to manage comfort and care. This might involve hiring specialized caregivers or coordinating with hospice services for end-of-life care.

Choosing the right option is deeply personal, requiring consideration of medical needs, personal preferences, and the values held dear by your loved one.

Making Informed Decisions

Navigating end-of-life care decisions is perhaps one of the most challenging aspects of dementia caregiving. Here are some steps to approach it with sensitivity and respect:

- Review Advanced Directives: If available, these documents provide invaluable insight into your loved one's wishes, offering guidance on decisions ranging from medical interventions to the preferred setting for care.
- Consult with Medical Professionals: Their insights can help clarify the implications of different care choices, ensuring decisions align with your loved one's health status and care needs.
- Family Discussions: Engage in open, honest conversations with family members. While not always easy, these discussions can ensure that everyone is on the same page and that decisions reflect collective values and respect for your loved one's wishes.

Legal and Ethical Considerations

End-of-life care also brings legal and ethical considerations to the forefront. Here's a look at some key aspects:

- Advance Directives and DNR Orders: These legal documents specify wishes regarding medical treatment and interventions. Ensuring they are up-to-date and readily available to healthcare providers is crucial.
- Ethical Considerations in Care Decisions: Balancing quality of life with medical interventions often involves ethical considerations. Engaging in discussions with healthcare providers, ethicists, or spiritual advisors can provide clarity and support in making these complex decisions.

Navigating the final stages of dementia gracefully involves a delicate balance of practical planning, heartfelt conversations, and informed decision-making. It's about ensuring that our loved ones' twilight days are marked by dignity, comfort, and respect for their wishes. Just as the golden hour casts a beautiful, serene light on the world, so too can our care and decisions illuminate the final chapter of our loved ones' lives with warmth and love.

Palliative Care: Comfort and Quality in the Final Days

At its core, palliative care is about enriching the quality of life for individuals facing the complexities of serious illness. It affirms life, emphasizing relief from discomfort and stress rather than leaning towards cure-oriented treatments. This care model thrives on a multidisciplinary approach, combining the expertise of healthcare professionals, spiritual advisors, and counselors to address physical symptoms and emotional and spiritual needs. The guiding principle here is to provide a blanket of care that shelters the individual and their loved ones, ensuring their journey is marked by dignity and respect.

Pain Management

As dementia progresses into its final stages, managing discomfort becomes the foremost priority. The goal is to ensure our loved ones remain as comfortable as possible, utilizing a tailored approach to pain management that considers their medical history and current condition. Based on the symptoms of a particular case, the pain management strategies may include:

- Medication: Utilizing pain relief options that align with the individual's needs and current health status, always aiming for the minimal effective dose to mitigate discomfort without unnecessary side effects.
- Non-Medical Interventions: Incorporating massage, aromatherapy, or music therapy can offer additional layers of

comfort, engaging the senses in a soothing, non-invasive manner.

- Environmental Adjustments: Creating a calming environment, free from loud noises and harsh lights, can significantly reduce stress and discomfort, promoting a sense of peace and well-being.

Emotional and Spiritual Support

Acknowledging the emotional and spiritual dimensions of this stage is vital. Palliative care teams place tremendous value on offering support that resonates with the individual's and family's belief systems and values. This might involve:

- Counseling Services: Providing access to counselors or therapists who can offer a space for individuals and families to express their fears, hopes, and emotions freely.
- Spiritual Care: For those who draw strength from their faith or spirituality, chaplains or spiritual advisors can offer guidance, prayer, or a listening ear, aligning with the family's beliefs and preferences.
- Memory Sharing: Encouraging families to share memories, stories, or cherished moments can be a powerful way to connect, celebrate the individual's life, and find comfort in shared experiences.

Working with Palliative Care Teams

Building a collaborative relationship with the palliative care team enhances the care experience, ensuring that your loved one's needs and wishes are at the forefront of care planning. You can do this by keeping the lines of communication with the care team open and transparent. Share insights about your loved one's preferences, personality, and life story to inform their care approach. You can also participate in care meetings, engaging in regular discussions about care goals, pain management strategies, and any adjustments in care plans to ensure that the care provided aligns with your loved one's needs and wishes. And finally, you must stay informed. Learning about the nature and benefits of palliative care can help you advocate more effectively for your loved one, ensuring they receive the care that best suits their needs.

In this sensitive time, palliative care embraces the belief that every moment of life is valuable. It offers a holistic approach that honors the individual's life journey, providing a foundation of support that encompasses physical comfort, emotional well-being, and spiritual peace. Through this care model, families find a compassionate ally, guiding them through the final days with grace, dignity, and profound respect for the life being honored.

Saying Goodbye: The Importance of Closure

In the quiet spaces of our hearts, where love and sorrow intertwine, the act of saying goodbye holds a sacred place. It's a moment that, despite its inherent sadness, can be filled with beauty, love, and profound respect. Here, we explore ways to navigate this delicate time, ensuring that farewells are as meaningful as the lives they honor.

Facilitating Goodbyes

Creating opportunities for meaningful farewells allows family members and friends to express their love, gratitude, and even apologies, fostering a sense of peace and closure for all involved. Consider these approaches:

- Private Moments: Arrange for private time between your loved one and each visitor. These quiet moments can be precious, offering space for personal words and gestures of love.
- Group Gatherings: If appropriate, a small gathering of close family and friends can be a beautiful way to share memories

and express collective gratitude for the life lived. Ensure it's a comfortable, familiar setting for your loved one.

- Memory Sharing: Encourage visitors to share their favorite memories or what they've admired about your loved one. Collecting these stories can be a powerful reminder of the impact your loved one has had on others' lives.
- Letter Writing: For those who cannot visit or find speaking difficult, letters are a tangible expression of love and farewell. Reading these to your loved one can be incredibly moving and meaningful.

Cherishing the Moments

In the final days, focusing on the value of presence—simply being with your loved one—can be incredibly comforting for you and them. Here are ways to cherish these fleeting moments:

- Comforting Touch: Holding a hand, gently stroking their hair, or a soft embrace can convey love and comfort without needing words.
- Peaceful Environment: Create a calm atmosphere with soft lighting, quiet music, or any ambient sounds your loved one enjoys. This tranquil setting can make the final moments together serene and comforting.
- Being Present: Sometimes, sitting quietly together, breathing in sync, can be a powerful way to connect. Let conversations flow naturally, without forcing them, and embrace the silence as a form of companionship.

Preparing for the Moment of Passing

The moment of passing, while deeply emotional, can also bring a sense of peaceful closure. Preparing yourself and your family can help ease the transition:

Memorial Services

Planning a memorial service that reflects the unique personality and wishes of your loved one ensures that those gathered not only mourn their loss but also celebrate the life they led. Consider these aspects:

- Venue Selection: Pick a place that holds special meaning for your loved one, be it a favorite park, their home, or a place where they loved to spend time, to add a personal touch to the service.
- Personalized Ceremonies: Tailor the service to include elements they love, like their favorite music, readings, or even a display of their artwork or crafts. This personalization turns the service into a heartfelt celebration of who they were.
- Memory Sharing: Encourage attendees to share their memories or stories, creating a tapestry of shared experiences that highlight the impact your loved one had on those around them.

Personal Memorials

Creating a space or item dedicated solely to remembering your loved one can offer solace during times of grief and serve as a tangible link to their memory. While you know best how you would like to remember your loved one, here are a few suggestions:

- Memory Books: Compile a book filled with photos, stories, and tokens representing significant moments in their lives. Inviting friends and family to contribute their memories can be a collaborative effort.
- Garden Memorials: Planting a tree or a garden in their honor serves as a living tribute that grows and flourishes over time, symbolizing the ongoing nature of their legacy.
- Custom Jewelry: Having a piece of jewelry made, perhaps incorporating something they cherished, like a stone from a

favorite ring or a snippet of their handwriting, keeps their memory close in a profoundly personal way.

Continuing Their Impact

Our loved ones' passions and contributions to the world around them need not end with their passing. Here are ways to ensure their influence continues to resonate:

- Advocacy and Awareness: If they are passionate about a particular cause, continuing to advocate in their name keeps their spirit of change alive. This could involve fundraising, awareness campaigns, or volunteer work related to their cause.
- Supporting Dementia Research: Contributing to dementia research in their name not only honors their battle but also aids in the quest for understanding and potentially curing the disease. Donations, fundraising events, or participating in awareness walks can all contribute to this cause.
- Legacy Projects: Initiating projects encapsulating their values or dreams contributes to a lasting legacy. Whether it's a community program, an art installation, or a published collection of their writings or recipes, these projects carry their essence into the future.

The Caregiver's Path After Loss

The road after losing someone dear, especially to an enveloping condition like dementia, stretches out, filled with reflections of the past and shadows of what was. It's a path that demands we tread softly, giving ourselves permission to grieve, mend, and, eventually, discover a renewed sense of purpose and connection.

Dealing with Grief

In its many layers, grief can envelop you like a dense fog, making the days blend into one another, each moment tinged with the memory of loss. While we may know the five stages of grief, it still feels like your heart is going to burst with pain. There is no proper way to get past it quickly, but there are a few steps to aid you in your healing:

- Acknowledging your grief: Allow yourself the space and grace to experience the full spectrum of emotions that come with loss. It's a sign of the deep love and connection you shared.
- Setting aside time for reflection: Dedicating moments in your day to sit with your memories and let them wash over you can be a healing practice. It could be looking through photos, visiting a place you both loved or simply sitting quietly with your thoughts.
- Writing as a form of release: Penning your thoughts, memories, and feelings can articulate and process your grief. Letters to your loved one, journal entries, or even poems can become valuable to your healing journey.

Self-Care and Healing

The intensity of caregiving doesn't leave quickly. Its echoes can linger, making it essential to consciously step into a space of healing and self-care. This includes:

- Prioritizing your health: Regular check-ups, nutritious meals, and restorative sleep are fundamental as you begin to rebuild your strength.
- Finding solace in nature: The rhythm of the natural world, its cycles of renewal and growth, can offer profound comfort and a reminder of the beauty that persists.
- Embracing activities that bring joy: Reconnecting with hobbies and interests set aside during your caregiving days can rekindle joy and spark creativity.

Finding a New Purpose

In the aftermath of loss, the world can feel untethered, as if a part of your identity has drifted away. Anchoring yourself again might mean:

- Exploring new or dormant passions: The time that opens up in the absence of caregiving duties presents an opportunity to explore interests that resonate with your current state.
- Giving back: Volunteering, particularly in ways that honor your loved one's memory or contribute to the fight against dementia, can offer a sense of purpose and connection.
- Learning and growing: Pursuing education, whether it's formal classes or informal learning experiences, can stimulate your mind and spirit, opening new paths for exploration and fulfillment.

Support Networks

The journey of healing is not one to walk alone. Surrounding yourself with understanding souls can feel like there's someone you can share your burden with. This reminds me of Dame Cicely Saunders' moving remark: "Suffering is only intolerable when nobody cares." So, please know that you are not alone, and you can find company in:

- Bereavement groups: Connecting with others who have experienced similar losses can provide comfort and understanding. Sharing stories and strategies for coping can lessen the weight of grief.
- Professional counseling: Sometimes, the complexity of our emotions and experiences requires the guidance of a professional. Therapists or counselors specializing in grief can offer valuable support and tools for navigating your feelings.
- Community resources: Libraries, community centers, and religious organizations often offer programs and services for those dealing with loss. These can be sources of comfort, education, and companionship.

Remember that healing is not a linear process. It weaves through moments of sorrow and glimpses of joy, through memories that ache and those that comfort. Allowing yourself the time and space to grieve, care for your well-being, seek out new horizons, and lean on the support of others is not just a pathway to healing—it's a testament to the resilience of the human spirit and the enduring power of love.

As we close this chapter, not just in the book but in the chapters of our own lives that we've shared with our loved ones, we carry forward the lessons learned, the love shared, and the strength garnered. The journey ahead, though uncertain, is ripe with the potential for growth, discovery, and the continuation of the love that has shaped us. And so, we step forward into the light of a new day with open hearts and the courage to embrace whatever comes next.

CHAPTER 11

VOICES FOR CHANGE

"You gain strength, courage, and confidence by every experience in which you really stop to look fear in the face. You must do the things which you think you cannot do." — Eleanor Roosevelt.

O nce you have experienced the presence of dementia and the loss that it brings, your life is altered forever. There is no way to return to who you used to be or to unlearn so many lessons that the hardships taught you. Life after this seeks fulfillment and meaning. For many, that comes from advocating for dementia care, early diagnosis, prevention, and possible treatments. Advocacy in dementia care involves changing currents, influencing policies, and navigating through uncharted waters to improve lives. It's about raising our voices for those we care for and future generations facing dementia's challenges.

For me, this chapter is a call to action; for you, it might be an inspiration. I aim to empower caregivers and communities to become advocates for change, ensuring that every individual with dementia receives the care, dignity, and respect they deserve.

Empowerment Through Advocacy

The power of one voice can echo through halls of legislation, across digital platforms, and within local communities, sparking change and inspiring action. With their firsthand experience, caregivers hold a unique perspective on the gaps and needs within the dementia care system. By turning these insights into advocacy, caregivers can push for improvements in care practices, funding for research, and the creation of supportive environments for individuals with dementia and their families.

- Where to Start: Identify issues you're passionate about, whether it's increasing funding for dementia research, improving caregiver support programs, or enhancing the quality of care in facilities. Begin by educating yourself on these topics and understanding the current landscape, challenges, and necessary changes.
- Local Community Centers and Government: Engage with local community centers to organize awareness events or workshops. Attend town hall meetings to discuss dementia care needs with local officials. These initiatives can lay the groundwork for broader change, starting from your backyard.

Starting Small

Every monumental change begins with a single step. Advocacy doesn't require grand gestures; small, consistent actions can accumulate, creating ripples that become waves of change. You can start by volunteering for local dementia care organizations or participating in community events to raise awareness. Use these platforms to share information and connect with others interested in making a difference. You may also host or organize workshops in community centers or libraries to educate the public about dementia, care needs, and how they can support advocacy efforts—partner with healthcare professionals or advocacy groups to provide comprehensive information.

Joining Forces

There is strength in numbers. By joining or forming advocacy groups, caregivers can amplify their voices, share resources, and coordinate efforts to effect change more effectively. Look for national or local advocacy groups focused on dementia care. These organizations often have resources, tools, and established networks that can help magnify your efforts. If there aren't existing groups in your area, consider starting one. Use social media platforms to connect with others in your community who share your passion for improving dementia care. Organize regular meetings to discuss strategies, share updates, and plan advocacy actions.

Effective Advocacy Strategies

Effective advocacy involves clear communication, strategic planning, and leveraging various platforms to reach stakeholders and policymakers.

- Communicating with Policymakers: When reaching out to policymakers, be clear, concise, and specific about the changes you advocate for. Personal stories can be powerful; share your experiences to illustrate the impact of current policies and the need for change.
- Social Media Campaigns: Utilize social media to raise awareness and garner support. Create engaging content that educates the public about dementia and the importance of your advocacy efforts. Use hashtags to increase visibility and encourage others to share your message.
- Awareness Campaigns: Organize events or campaigns during Alzheimer's & Brain Awareness Month or other relevant times of the year. Collaborate with local businesses, schools, and healthcare facilities to spread the word and engage the broader community in your efforts.

Through these strategies and actions, caregivers and community members can become powerful advocates for change in dementia care. It's about using our voices, experiences, and collective power to create a future where individuals with dementia and their caregivers are supported, valued, and respected.

Dementia-Friendly Communities: How to Get Involved

Creating a community that embraces and supports individuals with dementia and their families is not just a noble goal—it's an achievable one. The concept of a dementia-friendly community is rooted in understanding, respect, and action. These communities are designed to lift the fog of isolation and misunderstanding that often surrounds those living with dementia, providing a network of support that fosters independence and quality of life.

A Closer Look at Dementia-Friendly Initiatives

Imagine a place where every shop owner, police officer, and neighbor understands the challenges faced by individuals with dementia. In such a community, businesses have simple signage and layouts that reduce confusion, public transportation accommodates the unique needs of those with cognitive impairments, and social events are designed to be inclusive and accessible. The benefits of these initiatives extend beyond the individuals directly affected by dementia, creating a culture of empathy and support that enhances the entire community.

- Accessibility and Safety: A key focus is making public spaces and services more accessible and safer for individuals with dementia, reducing risks and barriers that might limit their independence.
- Informed Public Services: Training for first responders and public service workers ensures they can effectively and compassionately assist individuals with dementia, recognizing the signs and knowing how to respond.

- Supportive Social Networks: Encourages the formation of support groups and social gatherings that welcome individuals with dementia and their caregivers, fostering a sense of belonging and community.

Steps for Local Involvement

Anyone can contribute to the development of a dementia-friendly community. Here are practical ways to begin making a difference in your area:

- Educate Yourself and Others: Start by learning more about dementia and what it means to be dementia-friendly. Share this knowledge with friends, family, and colleagues to spread awareness.
- Connect with Local Leaders: Reach out to local government officials, community leaders, and business owners to discuss the importance of becoming dementia-friendly. Offer resources and ideas on how they can make a difference.
- Volunteer: Many communities have existing initiatives that could use your help. Whether assisting with a local memory café, participating in dementia awareness events, or helping to train volunteers, your time and effort can have a significant impact.

Working Together

The strength of a dementia-friendly community lies in its collective effort. Collaboration between businesses, healthcare providers, and public services creates a comprehensive support system that addresses the varied needs of individuals with dementia. Here are ways these collaborations can take shape:

- Partnerships with Local Businesses: Encourage businesses to adopt dementia-friendly practices, such as creating quiet shopping hours, training staff on how to assist customers with dementia, and simplifying store layouts and signage.

- Engagement with Healthcare Providers: Work with local healthcare providers to ensure they're aware of community resources and support networks available for their patients with dementia.
- Collaboration with Public Services: Advocate for public transportation options that cater to the needs of individuals with dementia, including training for drivers and conductors on assisting passengers with cognitive impairments.

Glimpse of a Positive Change

Across the globe, communities have embraced the dementia-friendly movement with inspiring results. You can also make a difference with your efforts; it doesn't matter where you come from. Your advocacy can lead to positive collective action from small to large cities. Just imagine:

- A small town envisions a comprehensive program aimed at training over 1,000 residents and business owners to become dementia-friendly. This visionary initiative leads to the creation of a network of safe spaces where individuals with dementia can confidently seek assistance if they ever feel disoriented or perplexed.
- In a bustling metropolis, public transportation services join forces with dementia advocacy groups to develop innovative strategies. Together, they train staff and implement dementia-friendly policies, revolutionizing the cityscape to ensure seamless and secure navigation for individuals with dementia.

Imagine a world where a chain of supermarkets pioneers a groundbreaking concept: "slow checkout lanes" staffed by empathetic employees specially trained to identify and aid customers with dementia. This imaginative initiative reduces stress and transforms the shopping experience into a positive and inclusive one for all.

If such initiatives have not yet been taken in your town or city, it is your chance to make them possible. This is your call to action and your inspiration. Wouldn't it be wonderful if we made the world more convenient for all our loved ones with dementia?

The Power of Storytelling

In the tapestry of human experience, stories hold a unique place. They carry the weight of emotions, the depth of understanding, and the power to connect across divides. For caregivers navigating the complex world of dementia, sharing their stories becomes a beacon of light for others in similar situations. Through these narratives, a profound sense of empathy and solidarity emerges, forging connections that transcend the challenges of dementia care.

Emotional Resonance

The impact of personal stories in the realm of dementia care cannot be overstated. Each narrative, rich with the intricacies of love, loss, and resilience, resonates deeply with listeners and readers alike. This emotional echo fosters a profound sense of empathy, bridging gaps in understanding and bringing to light the shared humanity among caregivers, individuals living with dementia, and the broader community. In sharing these stories, caregiving's often invisible struggles and triumphs are illuminated, fostering a deeper appreciation for the journey and the strength required to navigate it.

- Sharing Personal Triumphs and Trials: Recounting moments of breakthrough and bonding and the hurdles faced can offer solace and recognition to others on this path.
- Eliciting Empathy: By laying bare the emotional landscape of caregiving, stories can cultivate empathy among those unfamiliar with dementia, inviting them into the caregiver's world.

Platforms for Sharing

In today's digitally connected world, numerous platforms offer caregivers a space to share their stories. From the intimacy of blogs and social media to the collective sharing in support groups, each platform serves as a stage for these important narratives.

- Blogs and Personal Websites: Offer a personal space for in-depth storytelling, allowing caregivers to document their journey in a format that can evolve over time.
- Social Media Platforms: Shorter, more frequent updates on platforms like Instagram, Facebook, or Twitter can engage a broad audience, sparking conversations and connecting individuals across the globe.
- Local Support Groups: In-person or virtual meetings provide a communal space to share stories, offering immediate support and understanding from those in similar circumstances.
- Public Speaking and Workshops: Engaging in speaking opportunities at conferences, workshops, or community events can amplify the reach of these stories, touching hearts and minds in a live setting.

Writing as Therapy

Beyond its capacity to educate and connect, writing one's story serves as a powerful form of therapy. It's a process that allows for reflection, catharsis, and reclamation of agency in a journey often marked by uncertainty and loss. Putting experiences into words can help organize thoughts, process emotions, and find meaning amid challenges.

- Journaling: Keeping a daily journal can serve as a private outlet for emotions, offering a space to process the day-to-day experiences of caregiving.
- Blogging: Publicly sharing your journey can offer therapeutic benefits to the writer and extend support and understanding to readers navigating similar paths.

- Creative Writing: Exploring fiction, poetry, or memoir writing can allow caregivers to express their experiences in diverse and innovative ways, exploring the themes of caregiving, loss, and love through different lenses.

Inspiring Action

Perhaps one of the most potent outcomes of sharing the caregiving journey is the inspiration it provides to others. Stories can move people from empathy to action, whether through advocacy, volunteering, or becoming more informed about dementia and its impact.

- Motivating Volunteerism: Readers touched by personal stories may be inspired to volunteer their time with local dementia care organizations, support groups, or community projects.
- Driving Advocacy: Stories highlighting the challenges and gaps in dementia care can galvanize others to join advocacy efforts, pushing for changes in policy, funding, and social awareness.
- Educating and Informing: For some, these narratives serve as an introduction to the realities of dementia, inspiring a deeper dive into learning about the condition, its effects on families, and how society can offer better support.

In every shared story, there is an opportunity to touch a life, to kindle empathy, and to inspire action. The caregiving community finds its voice, strength, and capacity to effect change through these narratives. Whether through the written word, spoken tales, or the silent solidarity of shared experience, storytelling remains a vital tool in the journey of dementia care. It's a reminder that no one walks this path alone and that in the sharing, there is healing, understanding, and the power to inspire a brighter future for all touched by dementia.

Future of Dementia Care

In the evolving landscape of dementia care, light glimmers at the end of the tunnel, fueled by groundbreaking research and technological advancements. These strides promise a future where dementia care transcends traditional boundaries, offering more effective, compassionate, and tailored solutions.

Latest Research and Developments

In recent years, the scientific community has made significant leaps in understanding dementia. Researchers are unraveling the complex mechanisms behind cognitive decline, leading to the development of novel therapies aimed at slowing or even reversing the progression of dementia-related diseases. Among these are:

- Targeted Therapies: New treatments focus on specific biological targets, such as amyloid plaques and tau tangles, to halt their harmful effects on the brain.
- Genetic Insights: Genetic advances offer hope for personalized medicine approaches, identifying individuals at risk early and tailoring interventions to their specific genetic makeup.
- Preventative Strategies: A growing body of evidence points to lifestyle and environmental factors that can influence the risk of developing dementia. Research into these areas opens the door to prevention programs that could significantly reduce the incidence of dementia globally.

Technological Innovations

Technology is revolutionizing dementia care, offering tools that enhance quality of life, support caregivers, and provide innovative treatment options:

- Wearable Devices: From smartwatches that monitor health metrics to devices that track movement and predict potential falls, wearable technology is becoming an indispensable part of caregiving, offering peace of mind and promoting independence.

- Virtual Reality (VR): VR applications provide immersive experiences that can help with memory recall, relaxation, and even cognitive rehabilitation, transporting individuals with dementia to different times and places and stimulating their minds in a safe, controlled environment.
- Digital Platforms: Online platforms and apps facilitate better communication between caregivers, families, and healthcare providers. They offer resources, support networks, and management tools that streamline care coordination and information sharing.

The Role of Policy in Shaping Care

Policy changes play a critical role in shaping the future of dementia care. Advocacy efforts are pushing for policies that:

- Increase Funding: Direct more resources toward dementia research, care facilities, and support programs, ensuring that practical applications and accessible care options match the strides made in understanding and treating dementia.
- Support Caregivers: Implement policies that recognize the vital role of caregivers, providing them with financial support, resources, and training to ensure they can continue to provide care without sacrificing their well-being.
- Promote Early Diagnosis: Encourage healthcare systems to prioritize early detection and diagnosis of dementia, enabling timely intervention and access to care and support services.

A Vision for the Future

Envisioning the future of dementia care, we see a world where care is not only about managing symptoms but enhancing the dignity, independence, and joy of those living with dementia. This future is characterized by:

- Person-Centered Care: Tailored care plans that consider the individual's history, preferences, and needs, ensuring they remain at the heart of all care decisions.
- Accessibility: Care and support services that are universally accessible, removing barriers to care and ensuring everyone affected by dementia can benefit from advancements in treatment and technology.
- Comprehensive Support: A holistic approach to care that addresses medical needs and the emotional, social, and practical challenges faced by individuals with dementia and their caregivers.

As we look toward this horizon, hope and determination fuel our efforts. The advances in research, technology, and policy not only promise to transform dementia care but also offer a testament to the power of innovation, advocacy, and community in overcoming the challenges of dementia.

The strides we're making today lay the groundwork for a future where dementia care is more effective, compassionate, and tailored to the needs of each individual. It's a future where caregivers are supported, technology enhances care and connection, and policies reflect the urgent need for progress in dementia care.

As we move into the next chapter, let's carry the lessons learned, the advancements made, and the vision for a future where everyone with dementia is met with the care, respect, and dignity they deserve.

CHAPTER 12
REVIEW AND RESOURCES

"Caregiving often calls us to lean into love we didn't know was possible." - Tia Walker.

L et us take a moment before we begin this chapter to honor the courage, sincerity, and generosity you pour into your daily caregiving. It brings out the most deeply felt emotions and calls on every bit of strength to work to give the care our loved ones deserve. And yet, after giving everything you can, there is a persistent guilt and melancholy that accompanies the loss that dementia brings. Safe to say, it will never be easy, yet you continue to do your best. Part of this best is you reading this book, striving to get better each day.

In the hardships of caregiving, you need the right tools—a compass, a map, perhaps a friendly guide. Therefore, this chapter is designed to be just that for caregivers: a collection of essential resources, practical advice, and digital companions that light the way, offering support and direction when the path gets tough. You may also read it as a book revision and use it as a summary.

Resources and Guides

Let me begin by sharing some crucial resources that will surely be your companions on your caregiving journey. From books to software applications and online platforms, we never know what might be the answer to our roadblocks in caregiving. So, allow me to share a few with you so you can further explore the intricacies of caregiving.

Curated Reading List

Books are like lanterns in the dark, illuminating paths previously unseen. For those caring for someone with dementia, certain reads can offer not just light but companionship. Here's a list worth exploring:

- "The 36-Hour Day" by Nancy L. Mace and Peter V. Rabins: A go-to guide that covers the spectrum of caregiving, from medical advice to dealing with the emotional toll.
- "Creating Moments of Joy Along the Alzheimer's Journey" by Jolene Brackey Focuses on the power of creating joyful moments for those with Alzheimer's.
- "Dementia Reimagined: Building a Life of Joy and Dignity from Beginning to End" by Tia Powell: Offers a refreshing look at dementia care, emphasizing dignity and joy.
- "Loving Someone Who Has Dementia" by Pauline Boss: Explores the concept of ambiguous loss and offers strategies for coping with the grief that comes with dementia caregiving. These books provide guidance and remind us we're not alone on this journey.

Online Platforms

The internet is a forest in its own right, teeming with information. Yet, not all sources are created equal. Here are some websites that stand as beacons for caregivers:

- Alzheimer's Association (alz.org): Offers comprehensive information on dementia, a 24/7 helpline, and a community resource finder.
- The Caregiver Space (thecaregiverspace.org): A platform for caregivers to find support, share stories, and access resources.
- Dementia Care Central (dementiacarecentral.com): Provides educational articles, care strategies, and tips for financial planning.
- Age UK (ageuk.org.uk): Though UK-based, this site offers invaluable advice on care, health, and support services that are relevant globally. Navigating these sites can help you find local support groups, up-to-date research, and strategies to manage daily caregiving challenges.

App Selection

In today's digital age, your smartphone can be a versatile tool in your caregiving kit. Here are some apps that offer practical help:

- MyTherapy: Not just a medication reminder, this app also tracks mood, physical health, and has a diary feature for noting symptoms or changes.
- Alzheimer's Caregiver Buddy: Developed by the Alzheimer's Association, it provides care tips, stress management tools, and activities to engage your loved one.
- Lotsa Helping Hands: Ideal for coordinating care among family and friends, this app helps organize tasks, from meal delivery to doctor's appointments.
- MindMate: Offers stimulating games aimed at boosting cognitive skills, along with nutrition advice and workout routines suited for older adults. Apps like these can simplify aspects of caregiving, from medication management to creating stimulating activities for your loved one.

Navigating Information

Discerning reliable from misleading can be daunting with a wealth of information available. Here are some tips:

- Check the credentials of the author or organization providing the information. Trusted sources often have expertise in healthcare or direct experience in dementia care.
- Look for recent information. Dementia research is evolving, and strategies recommended a few years ago might have been updated.
- Cross-reference information. See if other reputable sources echo this guidance if you find a caregiving tip or medical advice.
- Be wary of quick fixes. Dementia is a complex condition, and solutions claiming to be miraculous cures are red flags.

Developing Your Care Plan: Templates and Checklists

Navigating the day-to-day responsibilities and unexpected challenges of caring for someone with dementia requires not just love and patience but a well-thought-out plan. A care plan acts like a roadmap, offering direction on daily tasks, medical appointments, and personal care routines, ensuring no detail is overlooked. Here, we'll explore how to craft a care plan that addresses the immediate needs and anticipates the journey ahead.

The Significance of a Detailed Care Plan

A detailed care plan brings clarity and structure to the often unpredictable nature of dementia care. It serves multiple purposes: ensuring consistent care, easing the handover between caregivers, and providing a reference point for medical professionals involved in your loved one's care. Furthermore, it can be a vital tool in emergencies, offering quick access to crucial information.

Templates for Success

Crafting a care plan from scratch might seem daunting. This is where templates and checklists come into play. They serve as a starting point, ensuring you cover all essential aspects of care:

- Personal Information: Full name, date of birth, medical ID, and contact information of your loved one.
- Medical Details: A list of diagnoses, medications (including dosages and schedules), allergies, and contact details for healthcare providers.
- Daily Routines: Meal times, preferred activities, and sleep schedules. Include personal care routines and any assistance required.
- Emergency Contacts: Names and numbers of family members, friends, and medical professionals to contact in case of an emergency.

Adapting these templates to fit your specific situation is key. Add sections as needed, such as dietary preferences, exercise routines, or behavioral management strategies.

Adaptability

Flexibility is crucial in a care plan. The progression of dementia means that needs and abilities will change over time. Regularly review and adjust your care plan to reflect these changes. This might mean altering medication schedules, introducing new activities, or updating emergency contacts. Keeping the care plan dynamic ensures it remains a relevant and effective tool.

Involving the Care Team

Caring for someone with dementia is rarely a one-person task. A collaborative approach ensures comprehensive care and allows for shared responsibilities. Involving family members, friends, and professionals in the care planning process ensures everyone is on the same page. Here's how to effectively engage your care team:

- Family Meetings: Regularly scheduled meetings with family members can help discuss updates, share responsibilities, and make collective decisions regarding care.
- Professional Input: Inviting healthcare providers to offer their expertise can ensure that the care plan aligns with medical advice and best practices.
- Task Delegation: Use the care plan to assign specific tasks to team members, such as medication management, appointment scheduling, or providing respite care.

In essence, a care plan is more than just a document; it's a living guide that evolves alongside the needs of your loved one. By starting with a solid template, maintaining flexibility, and fostering collaboration among the care team, you can create a personalized roadmap that supports not just the physical health of your loved one but their overall well-being.

Building Your Support Network

Navigating the path of a caregiver can sometimes feel like you're trying to move forward in dim light. Finding others to share the path with can not only brighten the way but can also offer invaluable guidance, comfort, and a sense of companionship. A robust support network is not just beneficial; it's a necessity for both you and your loved one with dementia. Here's how you can build and maintain these critical connections.

Identifying Potential Support

Spotting potential allies in your caregiving journey requires a keen eye and an open heart. Start close to home. Family members, friends, and neighbors often want to help but might not know how. Be clear about what support you need, whether it's someone to watch your loved one while you run errands or simply a friend to talk to when things get tough. Don't overlook the potential for support in broader circles, too. Colleagues, members of your religious community, or parents from your children's school can be unexpected sources of assistance and encouragement. Remember, people often appreciate the opportunity to lend a hand; they need to be asked.

The Power of Support Groups

Support groups are like lighthouses for caregivers navigating through storms. They offer a space to share experiences, exchange tips, and find solace in the understanding that you're not alone. Finding the right group might take a bit of research. Look for local chapters of national organizations, such as the Alzheimer's Association, which often host regular meetings. Online forums and social media groups can also provide flexible, accessible support. These platforms allow you to connect with others at any time, which can be particularly helpful during late-night hours when feelings of isolation can peak. Engaging with these groups can bring practical advice and emotional strength, reminding you that others understand your journey.

Creating a Care Circle

Think of a care circle as a constellation, with each star representing someone who brings a unique form of support. To assemble your constellation, consider the strengths and capabilities of each person in your network. Some might be good with hands-on care, while others excel at administrative tasks like scheduling or managing finances. Here are steps to creating an influential care circle:

- List potential members and their strengths.
- Organize a meeting, in person or virtually, to discuss your loved one's needs and how each person can contribute.
- Establish a schedule that rotates responsibilities, ensuring no one person becomes overwhelmed.

- Utilize group communication tools, like group chats or specialized apps, to keep everyone updated and allow for easy adjustments to the plan.

This approach divides the workload and fosters a shared commitment to your loved one's well-being, creating a more robust support network.

Maintaining Relationships

The demands of caregiving can strain even the strongest relationships. It's crucial to nurture these connections, ensuring they endure and flourish. Open communication is fundamental. Share your challenges and successes, and express gratitude often; recognition goes a long way in keeping relationships strong. Make time for one-on-one interactions with members of your support network, even if it's just a quick coffee or a brief phone call. These moments can reinforce your bonds and provide a much-needed break from the caregiving routine. Finally, be receptive to support in return. Allowing others to care for you strengthens mutual respect and understanding, reinforcing the foundation of your support network.

By now, you should know that building and maintaining a network of support is an ongoing process, one that adapts as the needs of your loved one change. Through each step, remember that reaching out for help is a sign of strength, not a weakness. By forging connections, sharing the load, and caring for your relationships, you illuminate the path for yourself and your loved one, ensuring you never walk in the dark.

Help Yourself

We are drawing near the end of this book, and I must share again that you cannot serve from an empty vessel. Prioritizing yourself is just as important as caring for your loved one. Acknowledge self-care as integral to caregiving and recognize its significance across physical, emotional, and spiritual dimensions. Physically, caregivers must prioritize regular exercise, nutritious eating habits, and sufficient rest to sustain their energy levels. Emotionally and mentally, managing stress through personalized techniques, seeking moments of joy, and accessing professional support is vital for preserving mental health amidst the challenges of caregiving, particularly when caring for someone with dementia. Spiritually, finding solace in practices like meditation, journaling, and connecting with nature is an anchor, nurturing a sense of peace and purpose throughout the caregiving journey.

Taking care of yourself is not a departure from your role as a caregiver —it's an integral part of it. Nurturing yourself allows you to share your best self with your loved one and navigate the caregiving path with strength and grace.

Let's carry with us the understanding that self-care is the foundation for effective caregiving. It's about ensuring we're as well-equipped as possible to meet the challenges and embrace the joys of supporting someone with dementia. With this mindset, we step forward, ready to explore further dimensions of caregiving, armed with knowledge, compassion, and a renewed commitment to our well-being.

Understanding Dementia Caregiving Challenges

Now that you've gained the insights to navigate the complexities of dementia care, it's time to share your newfound knowledge with others who are on the same journey.

By leaving your honest review of this book on Amazon, you'll guide other caregivers to the vital information they need and help continue the cycle of support and understanding.

Thank you for your contribution. The dementia caregiving journey is enriched when we share our knowledge—you play a crucial part in keeping this mission alive.

AFTERWORD

As we draw the curtains on this journey we've traversed together, I want to reiterate the core message of our shared narrative boldly. This book was conceived and crafted to empower you, the caregiver, as you navigate the intricate landscapes of dementia care. It has been an exploration into recognizing the multifaceted nature of dementia, fully embracing your invaluable role as a caregiver, understanding the critical importance of self-care, and preparing you for all stages of the caregiving journey.

We've journeyed through a 10-step guide designed to serve as your beacon through the foggy days and your anchor in turbulent waters. Together, we've delved into understanding dementia, building a compassionate and practical caregiving compass, enhancing communication, crafting a calm and nurturing environment, and preparing for the journey's end with dignity and love. These steps, these strategies we've discussed, are your toolkit, designed to empower you with hope, understanding, and actionable plans.

Reflecting on the emotional odyssey of caregiving, it's undeniable that this path is fraught with challenges that test your spirit, patience, and endurance. Yet, amidst these trials shines a remarkable resilience, a depth of love, and an undying hope that defines the essence of caregiving. Each chapter of this book has been a testament to the strength and love that caregivers like you embody daily.

Let this book not merely rest on your shelf but serve as a living resource for you. I encourage you to revisit its pages as you navigate the changing tides of your caregiving journey. Connect with support groups, advocate for better dementia care, and share your story to light the way for others. Remember, your voice, your experience, is a powerful beacon for those who walk this path alongside you.

Taking care of oneself is not selfish but a fundamental necessity. Your well-being is the wellspring from which compassionate and effective care flows. Nurturing your health, spirit, and peace is imperative to sustain the invaluable support you offer your loved one.

I urge you to stay informed and continue educating yourself about the latest dementia research and care strategies. Your advocacy and involvement are essential in shaping a future where dementia caregiving is recognized, respected, and supported by all facets of society.

In closing, from the depths of my heart, I thank you for your unwavering commitment to caregiving. Your journey is one of profound love and dedication, and it's my sincerest wish that this book serves as your companion, offering solace, guidance, and understanding. Let's envision a future where the dementia caregiving journey is illuminated by compassion, knowledge, and societal support. Thank you for being the beacon of hope and love in the lives of those you care for.

With deepest gratitude and respect,

Dean Ramsey

BIBLIOGRAPHY

National Institute on Aging. (n.d.). *Understanding different types of dementia.* https://www.nia.nih.gov/health/alzheimers-and-dementia/understanding-different-types-dementia

Terry, R. D., & Katzman, R. (2012). Plasticity in early Alzheimer's disease: An opportunity for intervention. *PMC.* https://www.ncbi.nlm.nih.gov/pmc/articles/PMC3419487/

National Institute on Aging. (n.d.). 12 myths about Alzheimer's disease. https://www.nia.nih.gov/health/alzheimers-and-dementia/12-myths-about-alzheimers-disease

California Department of Social Services. (n.d.). Ten tips for communicating with a person with dementia. https://www.cdss.ca.gov/agedblinddisabled/res/VPTC2/12%20Working%20With%20Consumers%20with%20Disabilities/Ten_Tips_Communicating_Dementia.pdf

Schulz, R., & Martire, L. M. (2013). Issues in dementia caregiving: Effects on mental and physical health, intervention strategies, and research needs. *PMC.* https://www.ncbi.nlm.nih.gov/pmc/articles/PMC3774150/

Mayo Clinic. (2021). Caregiver stress: Tips for taking care of yourself. https://www.mayoclinic.org/healthy-lifestyle/stress-management/in-depth/caregiver-stress/art-20044784

Salmon Health and Retirement. (n.d.). 7 benefits of caregiver support groups. Retrieved from https://salmonhealth.com/7-benefits-of-caregiver-support-groups/

AARP. (n.d.). Financial planning for dementia care: 9 tips. Retrieved from https://states.aarp.org/colorado/financial-planning-for-dementia-care-9-tips

Better Health Channel. (n.d.). Dementia - communication. Retrieved from https://www.betterhealth.vic.gov.au/health/conditionsandtreatments/dementia-communication

HelpGuide. (n.d.). Alzheimer's and dementia behavior management tips. Retrieved from https://www.helpguide.org/articles/alzheimers-dementia-aging/alzheimers-behavior-management.ht

Bennett, S., & Gaines, K. (2021). Use of technology and social media in dementia care. *PMC,* 12(1), 2047-2058. https://www.ncbi.nlm.nih.gov/pmc/articles/PMC8040150/

National Health Service (NHS). (n.d.). How to make your home dementia friendly. Retrieved from https://www.nhs.uk/conditions/dementia/living-with-dementia/home-environment/

Alzheimer's Association. (n.d.). Daily care plan. Retrieved from https://www.alz.org/help-support/caregiving/daily-care/daily-care-plan

A Place for Mom. (n.d.). 20 engaging activities for people with dementia at home. Retrieved from https://www.aplaceformom.com/caregiver-resources/articles/dementia-activities

Bibliography

Alzheimer's New Jersey. (n.d.). Managing challenging behaviors. Retrieved from https://www.alznj.org/resources/managing-challenging-behaviors/

National Health Service (NHS). (n.d.). How to make your home dementia friendly. Retrieved from https://www.nhs.uk/conditions/dementia/living-with-dementia/home-environment/

National Institute on Aging. (n.d.). Advance care planning: Advance directives for health care. Retrieved from https://www.nia.nih.gov/health/advance-care-planning/advance-care-planning-advance-directives-health-care

Alzheimer's Association. (n.d.). Financial and legal planning for caregivers. Retrieved from https://www.alz.org/help-support/caregiving/financial-legal-planning

Kaiser Family Foundation. (n.d.). Medicaid's role for people with dementia. Retrieved from https://www.kff.org/mental-health/issue-brief/medicaids-role-for-people-with-dementia/

Alzheimer's Association. (n.d.). Long-term care. Retrieved from https://www.alz.org/help-support/caregiving/care-options/long-term-care

Mayo Clinic. (2021). Caregiver stress: Tips for taking care of yourself. Retrieved from https://www.mayoclinic.org/healthy-lifestyle/stress-management/in-depth/caregiver-stress/art-20044784

Paller, K. A., Creery, J. D., Florczak, S. M., Weintraub, S., Mesulam, M.-M., Reber, P. J., ... & Maslar, M. (2018). Mindfulness training for people with dementia and their caregivers: Potential benefits and underlying mechanisms. *Frontiers in Psychology, 9*, 983. https://www.ncbi.nlm.nih.gov/pmc/articles/PMC6008507/

Alzheimer's Association. (n.d.). Support groups. Retrieved from https://www.alz.org/help-support/community/support-groups

mmLearn.org. (n.d.). Recognizing and coping with anticipatory grief. Retrieved from https://training.mmlearn.org/blog/recognizing-and-coping-with-anticipatory-grief

WebMD. (n.d.). 8 signs it's time for memory care. Retrieved from https://www.webmd.com/alzheimers/signs-time-memory-care

Alzheimer's Association. (n.d.). Choosing a residential care community. Retrieved from https://www.alz.org/media/documents/alzheimers-dementia-choosing-residential-care-ts.pdf

A Place for Mom. (n.d.). How to move a parent with dementia to assisted living. Retrieved from https://www.aplaceformom.com/caregiver-resources/articles/easing-transition-to-memory-care

DailyCaring. (n.d.). How to advocate for a loved one in long-term care: 7 smart steps. Retrieved from https://dailycaring.com/how-to-advocate-for-a-loved-one-in-long-term-care-7-smart-steps/

National Institute on Aging. (n.d.). End-of-life care for people with dementia. Retrieved from https://www.nia.nih.gov/health/end-life/end-life-care-people-dementia

Get Palliative Care. (n.d.). Palliative care and dementia: Deterioration of brain. Retrieved from https://getpalliativecare.org/whatis/disease-types/dementia-palliative-care/

Alzheimer's Association. (n.d.). Grief and loss as Alzheimer's progresses. Retrieved fromhttps://www.alz.org/help-support/caregiving/caregiver-health/grief-loss-as-alzheimers-progresses

Alzheimer's Disease International. (n.d.). Starting a self-help group. Retrieved from https://www.alzint.org/resource/starting-a-self-help-group/

Alzheimer's Disease International. (n.d.). Dementia friendly communities. Retrieved from https://www.alzint.org/what-we-do/policy/dementia-friendly-communities/

National Library of Medicine. (2023). Digital storytelling with persons living with dementia. *Journal of Applied Gerontology, 42*(5), 852–861. https://www.ncbi.nlm.nih.gov/pmc/articles/PMC10084455/

DelveInsight. (n.d.). Leading technology trends and innovations in dementia. Retrieved from https://www.delveinsight.com/blog/technological-innovations-in-dementia-care

DailyCaring. (n.d.). 12 best Alzheimer's and dementia books for caregivers. Retrieved from https://dailycaring.com/must-read-alzheimers-books-for-caregivers/

Alzheimer's Caregivers. (2023, December 5). 12 apps designed for people living with Alzheimer's disease and their caregivers. *Alzheimer's Caregivers.* https://alzheimerscaregivers.org/2023/12/05/12-apps-designed-for-people-living-with-alzheimers-disease-and-their-caregivers/

A Place for Mom. (n.d.). Dementia care plan: What to include at each stage. Retrieved from https://www.aplaceformom.com/caregiver-resources/articles/dementia-care-plan-by-stage

Alzheimer's Association. (n.d.). Building a care team. Retrieved from https://www.alz.org/help-support/i-have-alz/plan-for-your-future/building_a_care_team

www.ingramcontent.com/pod-product-compliance
Lightning Source LLC
Chambersburg PA
CBHW011835020426
42335CB00022B/2832